Wall Pilates Workouts

Strengthen Your Body with Pilates Exercises for Extraordinary Strength and Lasting Wellbeing

HOPE CARLSON

First Edition: August 2023

Copyright© 2023 HOPE CARLSON

Written by: HOPE CARLSON

This report aims to provide precise and robust information on the issue and the issue secured. The output could be rendered with the prospect of the manufacturer not needing to do bookkeeping, officially licensed or otherwise eligible administrations. Should an exhortation be relevant, lawful, or qualified, a rehearsed individual in the call should be required. The Statement of Principles was approved and endorsed by the American Bar Association Committee and the Publications and Associations Commission. It is not lawful to reproduce, copy, or distribute any portion of this study using either electronic methods or the community written. The registering of this delivery is deliberately disallowed, with the exception of written distributor authorisation, the ability of this material is not permitted. All resources are retained. The information provided is conveyed to be truthful and consistent, in so far as any chance, in the absence of thinking or something else, of any usage or misuse of any methods, procedures, or cookies found within is the special and definite responsibility of the receiver per user. Any civil duty or liability shall be put upon the seller for any reparation, damage, or money related misfortune attributable to the data received, whether explicitly or indirectly. Those authors assert all copyrights which the seller does not retain. The statistics herein are solely for instructional purposes and are all. The details were reached without consent or acknowledgement of guarantee. The markings used shall be without permission, and without the approval or help of the proprietor of the label shall be published. All logos and trademarks in this book are for information purposes only and are held explicitly by individuals who are not affiliated with this document.

LIMITED LIABILITY - DISCLAIMER:

The information provided in the book "Wall Pilates Workouts: Strengthen Your Body with Pilates Exercises for Extraordinary Strength and Lasting Wellbeing" is intended for general informational purposes only. The author and publisher have made every effort to ensure the accuracy and completeness of the content within this book; however, they make no representations or warranties of any kind, express or implied, regarding the completeness, accuracy, reliability, suitability, or availability of the information, products, services, or related graphics contained within for any purpose.

The use of the information provided in this book is at your own risk. The author and publisher shall not be liable for any loss, injury, or damage caused or alleged to be caused, directly or indirectly, by the information contained in this book.

It is essential to consult with a qualified healthcare professional or certified Pilates instructor before starting any new exercise program, including the Pilates exercises described in this book. Individual health conditions and physical abilities can vary, and what may be suitable for one person may not be appropriate for another. The author and publisher are not responsible for any injuries or health problems that may result from engaging in the exercises described in this book.

By reading and using the information provided in this book, you acknowledge that you are responsible for your actions and decisions concerning your health and fitness. You agree to release, indemnify, and hold harmless the author and publisher from any liability or responsibility for any injury or harm that may occur as a result of your use of the information in this book.

Always prioritize your safety and well-being. Listen to your body, and if you experience any discomfort, pain, or other adverse symptoms during the practice of Pilates exercises, discontinue the activity immediately and seek appropriate medical or professional advice. Your health and safety are of utmost importance, and this disclaimer is intended to ensure that you use the information provided in this book responsibly and wisely.

TABLE OF CONTENTS

INTRODUCTION 9

CHAPTER 1: INTRODUCTION TO PILATES AND THE CONCEPT OF WALL TRAINING (THE WALL) 13

    ORIGINS OF PILATES 13
    THE FUNDAMENTAL PRINCIPLES OF PILATES 16
    THE PAREDA (THE WALL) AS A KEY TOOL 18
    BENEFITS OF PILATES WITH THE PAREDA 20
    THE OBJECTIVES OF THE BOOK 23

CHAPTER 2: PILATES FUNDAMENTALS: ESSENTIAL PRINCIPLES FOR SUCCESS 26

    THE ORIGINS OF PILATES PRINCIPLES 26
    CONCENTRATION AS THE KEY TO SUCCESS 29
    CONTROL IN MOVEMENTS 31
    THE ROLE OF THE CORE (CENTER OF STRENGTH) 33
    SYNERGY AMONG THE PRINCIPLES 36

CHAPTER 3:" PRACTICAL PREPARATION: CREATING SPACE FOR YOUR WORKOUTS" 39

    DEFINING YOUR WORKOUT SPACE 39
    PILATES EQUIPMENT AND ACCESSORIES 41
    SAFETY AND COMFORT 44
    CREATING AN EFFECTIVE WORKOUT ROUTINE 47
    MINDSET AND AWARENESS 49

CHAPTER 4: "BASIC EXERCISES TO STRENGTHEN YOUR BODY WITH THE WALL" 53

    INTRODUCTION TO WALL EXERCISES 53
    EXERCISE 1: WALL SQUAT 55
    EXERCISE 2: WALL PUSH-UP 58
    EXERCISE 3: WALL PLANK 61
    EXERCISE 4: WALL STRETCHING 63

CHAPTER 5: "IN-DEPTH: ADVANCED EXERCISES TO CHALLENGE YOUR STRENGTH" 67

Introduction to Advanced Exercises 67
Exercise 1: Suspended Plank with the Wall Unit 69
Exercise 2: Inverted Roll-Up with the Wall Unit 72
Exercise 3: Leg Circle with the Wall Unit 74
Exercise 4: Swan Dive with the Wall Unit........................... 77

CHAPTER 6: CONTINUOUS FLOW: CREATING A PILATES WALL UNIT WORKOUT ROUTINE 81

Structuring Your Routine 81
Effective Sequences 83
Flexibility and Adaptability 86
Breathing and Flow 88
Maintaining Awareness... 91

CHAPTER 7: "FOCUS ON FLEXIBILITY: INCORPORATING STRETCHING INTO YOUR WORKOUTS" 95

The Importance of Stretching... 95
Types of Stretching... 97
Stretching Integration 100
Stretching and Relaxation.. 102
Development of a Stretching Routine 105

CHAPTER 8: "THE MENTAL SIDE OF PILATES: BALANCE AND MENTAL WELLBEING" 109

Mindfulness and Presence 109
Emotional Balance 111
Focus and Concentration 114
Stress Management... 116
Mind-Body Connection 119

CHAPTER 9: "COMBATING STRESS AND IMPROVING POSTURE WITH PILATES" 122

STRESS AND POSTURE 122
EXERCISES FOR RELAXATION 124
EXERCISES FOR POSTURE 127
BREATHING AND STRESS 130
STRATEGIES FOR WELL-BEING 133

CHAPTER 10: "SUPPORTING AN ACTIVE LIFESTYLE: INTEGRATING PILATES INTO YOUR DAILY ROUTINE" 137

IL PILATES AS A DAILY HABIT 137
MOMENTS OF AWARENESS 139
PILATES AT HOME 142
INVOLVING FAMILY AND FRIENDS 145
MAINTAIN VARIETY 148

CONCLUSION 152

Introduction

In the frenetic chaos of modern life, the quest for balance between physical and mental well-being has become an increasingly urgent priority. The accumulated tension from daily challenges can significantly impact our health and mood. In this context, the art of Pilates emerges as a beacon of hope, a path to strengthen the body and create lasting well-being. But let's go even further. Imagine discovering an extraordinary variant of this age-old practice: "Wall Pilates."

This book, "Wall Pilates Workouts: Strengthen Your Body with Pilates Exercises for Extraordinary Strength and Lasting Wellbeing," is a comprehensive guide for anyone wishing to explore the transformative benefits of Pilates using a surprising element: the wall. Through a series of innovative exercises and insights, we will take you on a journey to discover a new and captivating way to sculpt your body, develop extraordinary strength, and nurture lasting well-being.

Pilates as a Path to Well-being

To fully grasp the meaning of this book, we must start with the root of Pilates itself. Created by Joseph Pilates in the early 20th century, Pilates is a training system aimed at strengthening the body through the use of the mind. This unique practice focuses on awareness, breathing, and precise movements to create a balanced, flexible, and strong body. It has been described as "contrology" because it pits the mind against the body, leading to better muscle control and the elimination of tension.

But why "Wall Pilates"? The answer lies in the synergy created between the fundamental principles of Pilates and the support offered by a stable wall. This book will guide you through a series of exercises designed to use the wall as a key tool for muscle strengthening, flexibility improvement, and overall well-being promotion.

The Importance of Strength and Flexibility

Strength and flexibility are the foundations of our body. Adequate strength allows us to tackle daily physical challenges, while flexibility enables us to move freely and prevent muscle tension and injuries. "Wall Pilates" combines these two aspects into a single practice that aims to create a harmonious balance between strength and flexibility.

A Comprehensive Guide

This book is designed to be a comprehensive guide to "Wall Pilates." We will start from the beginning, guiding you through the origin of

Pilates and the fundamental principles that constitute its core. We will explore the crucial role of the "core" or centre of strength and the synergy between the principles that make it possible. You will be introduced to practical preparation, including defining your workout space, the necessary equipment, and measures to ensure safety and comfort during practice.

Once a solid foundation is established, we will dive into the basic exercises of "Wall Pilates." We will guide you through each movement, explaining its benefits and providing detailed instructions for safe and effective execution. You will learn how to develop a personalized workout routine and how to maintain the mindset and awareness necessary to get the most out of your practice.

But we won't stop there. You will also have the opportunity to explore advanced exercises that will challenge your strength and flexibility, taking you to new levels of skill and well-being. You will create fluid sequences of exercises that can be adapted to your needs and fitness level, always keeping your practice fresh and engaging.

A Journey Toward Your Best Self

This book is a key to unlocking your potential, creating a deeper connection between mind and body, and achieving extraordinary strength and mental well-being. "Wall Pilates" is an opportunity to challenge yourself, to create a lasting balance between physical strength and mental well-being. With commitment and dedication, you can embark on a transformational journey that will lead you to become the best version of yourself. Start this journey with us and discover how "Wall Pilates" can change your life in surprising ways.

Chapter 1: Introduction to Pilates and the Concept of Wall Training (The Wall)

Origins of Pilates

The origins of Pilates can be traced back to the early 20th century, and this discipline was developed by Joseph Hubertus Pilates, a man who left an indelible mark on the world of fitness and wellness. To fully grasp the evolution and significance of Pilates, it's necessary to take a step back in time and explore the roots of this discipline.

Joseph Pilates was born in Germany in 1883. From a young age, afflicted with various ailments such as asthma and rickets, he faced significant challenges in maintaining his health. However, these obstacles drove him to seek solutions to improve his physical condition. He began to study and draw from various exercise traditions, including yoga, gymnastics, and martial arts. This exploration led him to develop a set of fundamental principles that would eventually form the foundation of Pilates.

During World War I, Joseph Pilates was interned as a prisoner of war in a concentration camp. In this hostile environment, he continued to refine his ideas and exercises, creating a training system that could be practised by anyone, even in confined spaces. He began teaching his exercise techniques to fellow prisoners, contributing to their physical and mental well-being despite adverse circumstances.

After the war, Joseph Pilates moved to the United States, where he founded his studio in New York City in the 1920s. Here, he began teaching his method, which was then known as "Contrology." This name reflected Pilates' philosophy that total control of the body was essential for achieving health and wellness.

The Pilates method gradually spread in the 1930s and 1940s, attracting the attention of dancers, actors, and professional athletes. Joseph Pilates built a strong client base, including prominent figures from the entertainment and sports world. These individuals experienced the benefits of Pilates in the form of increased strength, flexibility, coordination, and an overall improvement in health and well-being.

One of the early famous supporters of Pilates was the dancer Martha Graham, who used the method to enhance her technique and endurance. The renowned dancer George Balanchine also became a follower of Pilates and encouraged his dancers to practice it to improve their performance.

In the 1960s, Pilates gained further visibility through books and articles promoting its benefits. This led to increased public interest in the method.

After Joseph Pilates' death in 1967, his method continued to be developed and adapted by his students and subsequent teachers. Pilates became a widely recognized and appreciated form of exercise, with millions of people worldwide practising it to enhance their physical and mental health.

In recent years, Pilates has been integrated into fitness programs, physical rehabilitation, and even high-level sports activities. Pilates studios have become widespread, offering classes tailored to various needs and skill levels. The versatility of Pilates, which can be practised on a mat or with specialized equipment, makes it suitable for a wide range of individuals, from beginners to professional athletes.

In conclusion, the origins of Pilates can be traced back to Joseph Pilates, a man who overcame significant personal challenges and developed a training system that revolutionized the approach to health and fitness. Today, Pilates is widely recognized as an effective method for improving strength, flexibility, and overall well-being, continuing to inspire and enhance the lives of many people worldwide.

The Fundamental Principles of Pilates

The fundamental principles of Pilates constitute the heart and soul of this fitness discipline. Developed by Joseph Pilates himself, these principles represent a philosophy of movement that goes beyond physical training. In the following paragraphs, we'll explore in detail the six fundamental principles of Pilates and how they influence the practice of this discipline.

1. Concentration: The first fundamental principle of Pilates is concentration. In Pilates, it's not enough to simply go through the motions mechanically. You must fully focus on each movement, how your body moves in space, and how muscles are engaged. This level of concentration not only enhances the effectiveness of the exercise but also helps develop a greater awareness of your own body.

2. Control: Control is another key principle of Pilates. It means having complete control over your body's movements during each exercise. This isn't just about muscle strength but also precision of

movement. In Pilates, the aim is to avoid abrupt or uncontrolled movements, emphasizing smooth and precise control.

3. Centering: The concept of the "center" is central in Pilates. It refers to the group of muscles in the lower abdominal, lumbosacral, and pelvic regions. This area, often called the "core," is considered the body's centre of strength. All Pilates movements originate from here, and their strengthening is crucial for better posture, improved stability, and increased overall strength.

4. Flow of Movement: Pilates emphasizes fluidity and continuity in movements. Exercises are designed to flow naturally from one to another without abrupt interruptions. This flow of movement not only makes exercises more effective but also contributes to a mind-body connection, allowing for a greater sense of well-being during practice.

5. Precision: Precision is an essential principle for reaping the maximum benefits from Pilates. It involves performing each movement with attention to detail and avoiding excessive or incorrect movements. This not only

enhances training effectiveness but also reduces the risk of injury.

6. Breath: Controlled breathing is a distinctive feature of Pilates. During exercises, deep and controlled breathing is encouraged, integrated with movement. This intentional breathing helps maintain concentration, support strength, and promote relaxation during the workout.

In addition to these six fundamental principles, Pilates also promotes stretching and flexibility as integral parts of the practice. The goal is to create long, supple muscles rather than bulky and contracted ones.

It's important to note that the fundamental principles of Pilates aren't limited to physical training but can be applied to everyday life. Concentration, control, and body awareness can help improve posture, prevent lower back pain, and enhance overall quality of life.

The Pareda (The Wall) as a Key Tool

The Pareda, also known as "The Wall" in the context of Pilates, is a key and innovative element within this fitness discipline. This tool offers a range of unique advantages that can transform the training experience and contribute to achieving better strength, flexibility, and overall well-being.

The Pareda is essentially a vertical wall or a solid and stable surface used as support during Pilates exercises. Its primary function is to provide a fixed reference point against which the practitioner can work to improve their posture, alignment, and endurance. This tool was originally designed by Joseph Pilates to offer extra support during exercises, allowing practitioners to focus on the precision of movements without worrying about balance.

One of the most common ways in which the Pareda is used in Pilates is to enhance spinal mobility. During stretching and lengthening exercises, the Pareda provides a stable anchor point that enables practitioners to achieve greater spinal extension, improving flexibility and posture. This is particularly beneficial for those experiencing tension in the upper back or neck.

The Pareda is also an excellent tool for building strength. During resistance exercises like planks or squats, the Pareda acts as a surface to push against or pull from, creating greater muscle challenge. This helps build stronger and more toned muscles throughout the body. Additionally, the Pareda can be used for specific abdominal strengthening exercises, aiding in the development of the body's core strength.

The Pareda also offers opportunities for balance and body control exercises. Movements involving leg lifts or body rotations can be performed with the support of the Parada to provide stability. This helps practitioners improve their balance and coordination, as well as develop a greater awareness of their body.

A particularly interesting aspect of using the Pareda is its adaptability for all fitness levels. Beginners can use it as support for basic exercises, while more advanced athletes can leverage it to further challenge themselves by creating more complex exercise variations.

Beyond the physical benefits, using the Pareda in Pilates also promotes greater body awareness. As practitioners work with the Pareda, they develop a deeper understanding of their posture, tension points, and areas that require more attention. This awareness can be applied to daily life, helping prevent pain and tension and maintaining better posture.

Benefits of Pilates with the Pareda
The benefits of Pilates with the Pareda are manifold and encompass a range of physical and

mental advantages that make this training practice a popular choice for many individuals. The use of the Pareda, or "The Wall," adds a unique and dynamic element to Pilates, offering a variety of benefits that contribute to overall improvement in strength, flexibility, and well-being.

One of the primary benefits of Pilates with the Pareda is the added support provided by this solid and stable surface during exercises. This support is particularly beneficial for beginners who are learning the basic movements of Pilates. The Pareda allows them to perform exercises with greater safety, reducing the risk of injuries and encouraging proper form. This is crucial as good form is essential for reaping the maximum benefits from Pilates training.

Another key advantage is the improvement in posture. Many Pilates exercises target the muscles of the core and upper back, helping to correct poor posture. The Pareda offers excellent support for performing exercises aimed at posture improvement, allowing the practitioner to focus on correcting their posture and body alignment. This is especially useful for those who spend long hours at a computer or suffer from tension in the upper back and neck.

Pilates with the Pareda also offers a greater variety of exercises and resistance options. This tool can be used to perform a wide range of exercises, from flexibility and stretching to resistance training. This means that the workout can be customized to suit the specific needs and goals of each individual. For example, you can adjust the angle of the Pareda to make exercises more or less challenging.

The Pareda is also an excellent tool for improving flexibility. During stretching and lengthening exercises, the Pareda provides a stable anchor point that helps the practitioner achieve greater muscle extension. This is particularly beneficial for those looking to enhance muscle flexibility, which can help prevent injuries and increase range of motion.

A fundamental aspect of Pilates with the Pareda is the opportunity to develop core strength. Exercises targeting the abdominal, lower back, and pelvic muscles can be performed using the Pareda as support. This helps build a solid foundation of core strength, which is essential for stability, balance, and improved posture.

Finally, Pilates with the Pareda can also contribute to mental well-being. The concentration required to perform exercises with precision, coupled with controlled breathing, promotes a sense of relaxation and mind-body connection. This can help reduce stress and enhance self-awareness.

The Objectives of the Book

The objectives of this book are diverse and ambitious. "Wall Pilates Workouts: Strengthen Your Body with Pilates Exercises for Extraordinary Strength and Lasting Wellbeing" aims to provide readers with a comprehensive and detailed guide to Pilates training using the Pareda. These objectives go beyond simply presenting a series of exercises; the book aims to inspire, educate, and guide readers on a journey of physical improvement and overall well-being.

First and foremost, the primary objective is to provide a clear understanding of the fundamental principles of Pilates and how they apply when using the Pareda. This means explaining concentration, control, the role of the "core" (the centre of strength), the fluidity of movements, precision, and breathing, and how these principles can be integrated into Pareda exercises.

Secondly, the book aims to provide readers with a wide range of specific Pilates exercises that can be performed with the Pareda. These exercises are described in detail, with clear instructions and illustrations to ensure that readers can perform them correctly and safely. The exercises are progressive, allowing practitioners to start at basic levels and progress to more advanced ones as they gain strength and confidence.

Another key objective is safety. The book provides important safety guidelines for Pareda training, including the correct use of equipment and injury prevention. Safety is of paramount importance in any form of training, and this book is committed to ensuring that readers can practice Pilates with the Pareda responsibly.

Additionally, the book promotes customization. Each individual is unique, with different needs and goals. Therefore, the goal is to provide readers with the tools to adapt exercises and Pilates training to their personal needs. This means that the book is not a "one-size-fits-all" solution but rather a resource that can be tailored to meet the specific needs of each individual.

An implicit objective is also to inspire and motivate readers. Pilates with the Pareda is a practice that requires commitment and dedication. The book offers success stories and testimonials from people who have benefited from Pilates, aiming to motivate readers to engage and maintain a consistent practice. Furthermore, it emphasizes the positive aspects and tangible results that readers can achieve through Pilates training.

Lastly, but no less important, the book's objective is to promote overall well-being. Pilates is not only a form of physical training but also a path to improving mental well-being and quality of life. The book encourages readers to consider Pilates as a tool to enhance their physical and mental health, promoting an active lifestyle and greater self-awareness.

In conclusion, "Wall Pilates Workouts: Strengthen Your Body with Pilates Exercises for Extraordinary Strength and Lasting Wellbeing" has a series of clear and ambitious objectives. This book aims to educate, inspire, and guide readers on their journey to better health and well-being through Pilates with the Pareda. Its mission is to offer a comprehensive and detailed guide that is accessible and useful to individuals of all fitness levels and experience, promoting a better quality of life through training and self-improvement.

Chapter 2: Pilates Fundamentals: Essential Principles for Success

The Origins of Pilates Principles

To fully understand the fundamental principles of Pilates, it is essential to explore their origins and the context in which they were developed. The principles that now form the foundation of this fitness discipline have their roots in the life experiences and influences of Joseph Hubertus Pilates, the founder of Pilates.

Joseph Pilates was born in Germany in 1883 and grew up in an era where health and fitness were significant concerns. From a young age, Pilates suffered from various health issues, including asthma and rickets. These health challenges drove him to seek solutions to improve his physical and mental well-being. This quest for health improvement led him to study and learn from various exercise traditions, including yoga, gymnastics, martial arts, and dance.

Joseph Pilates' influences were broad and diverse. During his learning journey, he drew inspiration from various disciplines. For instance, he studied yoga to gain a deeper understanding of the mind-body connection, breathing, and stretching. From gymnastics, he learned the importance of strength training and flexibility. Martial arts provided him with knowledge about discipline, body control, and endurance. Finally, from dance, he acquired expertise in fluid movement and grace in motion.

The combination of these influences and Joseph Pilates' personal experiences led to the creation of the fundamental principles that are now the bedrock of Pilates. These principles represent a holistic approach to training and health, aiming to develop not only physical strength but also mental awareness and overall well-being.

One of the most important fundamental principles is concentration. Joseph Pilates believed that body control should start with the mind. Concentration is crucial for executing each movement precisely and intentionally. This approach to concentration enhances the effectiveness of Pilates training, as each movement is performed with awareness and attention to detail.

Another crucial principle is control. Pilates taught his students to perform exercises with complete control of movement, avoiding abrupt or uncontrolled motions. This approach promotes not only safety during training but also strengthens the mind-body connection. Control allows for precise execution of exercises and injury prevention.

The third fundamental principle is the role of the "core" or the centre of strength. Pilates emphasized the importance of developing and strengthening the muscles of the abdomen, lower back, and pelvic area. These muscles are essential for stabilizing the body, improving posture, and preventing lower back pain.

Additionally, Pilates promotes the flow of movement. This means that exercises are designed to flow smoothly and without abrupt interruptions. This flow of movement not only makes exercises more effective but also helps create a mind-body connection, allowing for a greater sense of well-being during training.

Finally, the fifth fundamental principle is breathing. Pilates taught controlled breathing that integrated with movement. This deep and controlled breathing not only helps maintain concentration but also supports strength and relaxation during training.

In summary, the fundamental principles of Pilates have their roots in the experiences and influences of Joseph Pilates. These principles were developed to create a holistic approach to training that goes beyond mere physical fitness, also promoting the mind-body connection and overall well-being. They represent the foundation on which Pilates is built and are essential for reaping the maximum benefits from this fitness discipline.

Concentration as the Key to Success

Concentration is one of the fundamental pillars of Pilates, a key principle that emphasizes the importance of deep attention and mindfulness during training. It is considered a key to success as it directly influences the quality of exercises performed and the achievement of goals related to strength, flexibility, and overall well-being.

In the context of Pilates, concentration goes beyond the mere act of mechanically performing exercises. It involves directing attention deliberately and intentionally to every aspect of the movement. This entails a profound mind-body connection in which the mind guides the body through each exercise, constantly monitoring alignment, posture, and the precision of movements.

One of the reasons why concentration is considered so crucial is that Pilates is an activity that demands considerable precision. Many of the positions and sequences of movements involved require accurate control and coordination for correct execution. Without concentration, there is a risk of performing exercises incorrectly, reducing the effectiveness of the training and increasing the risk of injuries.

Moreover, concentration enables the development of greater body awareness. This means being able to perceive physical sensations, such as muscle tension, stretching, and stability while performing exercises. This awareness is essential for tailoring exercises to individual needs and detecting any tensions or imbalances in the body that require attention.

Concentration in Pilates goes hand in hand with controlled breathing. During exercises, breathing is a key element that helps maintain concentration. Deep and controlled breathing not only provides oxygen to the muscles in action but also helps maintain a steady rhythm and a continuous flow of movement. This synchrony between breathing and movement contributes to the effectiveness of the training.

Concentration in Pilates can also have a positive impact on the mind. Since it requires intense mental focus, practising Pilates can help free the mind from everyday stress and concerns. During the practice, one focuses exclusively on physical sensations and movements, creating a relaxing break from the hectic mind.

An important aspect to consider is that concentration in Pilates is a skill that can be developed and improved over time. Beginners may find it challenging to maintain concentration throughout an entire session, but with consistent practice, it becomes more natural. It is a learning process that reflects the central concept of Pilates: training both the body and the mind.

Control in Movements

Control in movements is one of the fundamental principles of Pilates and plays a crucial role in the practice of this fitness discipline. This principle emphasizes the importance of executing each exercise with total and deliberate control, avoiding abrupt or uncontrolled movements. Control is essential for maximizing the benefits of Pilates training and ensuring safety during exercise.

One of the primary reasons why control of movements is so essential in Pilates is its emphasis on precision. Pilates exercises often involve specific positions and movements that require a high degree of precision to be performed correctly. This precision is crucial for achieving the maximum benefits from exercises because even a small deviation from the correct form can reduce the effectiveness of training and increase the risk of injuries.

Control in movements is particularly evident during exercises like the "Teaser" or the "Hundred," where the practitioner must coordinate the movement of various parts of the body harmoniously and with control. These exercises demand a high level of strength, flexibility, and control to be successfully executed.

Furthermore, control is closely linked to controlled breathing in Pilates. Controlled breathing is another fundamental principle that seamlessly integrates with control in movements. During exercises, regular and controlled breathing helps maintain concentration and rhythm. This contributes to greater body awareness and the maintenance of proper form.

Control in movements is not only about precision but also contributes to strengthening the mind-body connection. Because the practitioner must be fully aware of what they are doing during each exercise, a deeper connection between the mind and body develops. This awareness enhances mental presence during training, creating a more meaningful and rewarding experience.

An interesting aspect of control in movements is that it extends well beyond Pilates training itself.

This principle can be applied in daily life. Awareness and control of movements can help improve posture, coordination, and safety during everyday activities, reducing the risk of injuries.

Maintaining control of movements requires constant practice and awareness. Beginners may find it challenging to maintain total control, but with time and experience, it becomes more natural. It is a learning process that reflects the gradual and progressive approach of Pilates, where practitioners start with basic exercises and advance as they develop strength and control.

In conclusion, control in movements is one of the fundamental principles of Pilates that defines its essence. This principle emphasizes precision, awareness, and safety in training, contributing to improved strength, flexibility, and overall well-being. Control is not only about the physical aspect but also promotes a greater mind-body connection and can be applied in daily life to enhance posture and coordination. In Pilates, control is the key to achieving tangible results and maintaining a safe and effective practice.

The Role of the Core (Center of Strength)

The role of the "core," or centre of strength, in Pilates is of fundamental importance and is one of the central principles of this fitness discipline.

The term "core" refers to a group of muscles that includes the abdominal muscles, lower back muscles, pelvic muscles, and diaphragm. These muscles form the core of the body and are essential for stabilizing, supporting, and coordinating movements.

In Pilates, the centre of strength is considered the body's energy centre. This area is responsible for supporting the spine, providing stability to the torso, and facilitating limb movement. In other words, the centre of strength is involved in virtually every action and movement of the body.

One of the primary goals of Pilates is to strengthen and develop the centre of strength. This is important for many reasons. Firstly, a strong core provides stability and support to the spine. This is crucial for maintaining proper posture and preventing back pain and injuries. When the core is weak, the spine is more vulnerable to strains and stresses, which can lead to long-term health issues.

Furthermore, a strong core is essential for efficient and coordinated movement. In daily movements and sports activities, the centre of strength acts as a bridge between the torso and the limbs. For example, during running, a strong core helps stabilize the upper body, allowing the legs to move with greater power and efficiency.

This enhances athletic performance and reduces the risk of injuries.

The role of the core in Pilates is evident in many of the specific exercises. During exercises like the "Roll-Up" or the "Hundred," the practitioner is called upon to actively engage the abdominal muscles to stabilize the torso and facilitate movement. These exercises aim to strengthen the core in a balanced way, involving both the upper and lower abdominal muscles.

In addition to strength, Pilates also aims to develop core flexibility. This means working on the range of motion of the abdominal and lower back muscles. Balanced core flexibility contributes to improved trunk mobility, which is crucial for maintaining proper posture and preventing muscle stiffness.

Another important aspect of the core's role in Pilates is the coordination of movements. Pilates promotes the integration of core muscles with breath control and movement control. This coordination is essential for executing exercises smoothly and controlled while maintaining mental focus during training.

In summary, the role of the core in Pilates is of vital importance. This principle is at the heart of the discipline and influences key aspects such as posture, stability, strength, flexibility, and coordination. Strengthening the core through Pilates training offers a range of benefits that go beyond mere physical fitness, enhancing the quality of life, preventing injuries, and promoting better performance in daily and sports activities. Ultimately, the core is the cornerstone of Pilates, helping to create a strong, balanced, and well-coordinated body.

Synergy Among the Principles

The synergy among the fundamental principles of Pilates is a crucial element that defines the very essence of this fitness discipline. Pilates is not based on isolated principles but on a set of interconnected principles that work synergistically to create a holistic approach to body training and overall well-being.

The synergy among the principles of Pilates is evident from the beginning of each session. Concentration is the starting point, as it requires a focused and attentive mind to guide the body through the exercises. This concentration leads to greater control in movements, where each action is executed deliberately and mindfully. Control, in turn, promotes safety during training, reducing the risk of abrupt or incorrect movements.

A fundamental component of the synergy among the principles is controlled breathing. Regular and controlled breathing not only provides the necessary oxygen to the active muscles but also helps maintain a steady rhythm and a constant flow of movement. This coordination between breathing and movement contributes to the effectiveness of the training and body awareness.

The role of the core (centre of strength) is central to this synergistic process. A strong and flexible core stabilizes the body during exercises, providing the foundation for controlled and fluid movements. Without core involvement, many Pilates exercises would lose their purpose and effectiveness. Additionally, a well-trained core also helps maintain proper posture, reducing the risk of back strains and pain.

The synergy among the principles of Pilates becomes even more evident in complex movements. Advanced exercises like the "Swan Dive" or the "Mermaid" require concentration, control, respiratory coordination, and core engagement in a single harmonious action. This synergistic integration of the principles creates a seamless sequence of movements that challenge the body in different ways, developing strength, flexibility, and coordination.

A fundamental aspect of the synergy among the principles is the mind-body connection. This is the heart of Pilates, where the mind guides the body through a series of controlled actions. This mind-body connection not only enhances the effectiveness of the exercises but also promotes a sense of well-being and relaxation during training.

Finally, the synergy among the principles is reflected in the consistent practice of Pilates. Over time and with regular practice, concentration, control, respiratory coordination, and core engagement become increasingly natural. The synergy among these principles becomes an integral part of the practitioner's approach to training and daily life.

In conclusion, the synergy among the fundamental principles of Pilates is what makes this discipline so unique and effective. These principles work together in harmony to promote physical and mental health, improving strength, flexibility, posture, and body awareness. This synergy creates a holistic approach to training that transforms not only the body but also the mind, promoting overall well-being and a balance between mind and body. In Pilates, the synergy among the principles is the key to achieving lasting results and establishing a profound connection with one's own body.

Chapter 3:" Practical Preparation: Creating Space for Your Workouts"

Defining Your Workout Space

Defining your workout space is a crucial step when embarking on a Pilates practice. Creating an appropriate and dedicated environment for your training can make the difference between an effective and satisfying practice and a fragmented or disorganized experience. In this chapter, we will explore the importance of defining a dedicated workout space for Pilates and provide practical tips on how to do so.

To begin with, it is essential to identify a quiet and distraction-free space. The atmosphere should be relaxing and free from noise or interruptions. Choose a location in your home or gym that allows you to fully concentrate on your practice without external interference. This workout environment should inspire tranquillity and focus.

A mat is often the starting point for defining your workout space. Make sure you have a quality mat to work on. This mat should be thick enough to provide adequate support for your body during exercises. The mat's surface should also be non-slip to ensure a stable foundation during practice.

If you are practising Wall Pilates (using the wall), consider the space needed to position it. Ensure there is enough clear space around the wall to perform exercises without obstacles. If possible, securely anchor it to the wall to prevent unwanted movement during practice.

Organize your space so that everything you need is easily accessible. Accessories like resistance bands, Pilates balls, and small equipment should be neatly positioned and within reach. This will prevent frequent interruptions during practice to search for necessary equipment.

A frequently overlooked aspect of defining the workout space is lighting. Ensure that your workout area is well-lit so that you can see clearly during exercises. Good lighting contributes to the safety and precision of movements.

Additionally, consider the surrounding environment. The temperature should be comfortable to avoid feeling too hot or too cold during practice. If space allows, consider using plants or decorative elements that add a personal touch to your workout environment.

A crucial aspect is the cleanliness and orderliness of your workout space. Keep the mat and equipment clean and organized. This creates a pleasant environment in which to train and motivates you to return regularly to practice.

Finally, when defining your workout space, take the time to personalize it according to your preferences. Add elements that inspire and motivate you. This may include music you enjoy listening to during practice, a motivational poster, or a scented candle to create a relaxing atmosphere.

In summary, defining the workout space in Pilates is a fundamental step in creating a supportive and motivating environment for your practice. Choose a quiet location, organize your equipment neatly, pay attention to lighting, and keep your space clean and inviting. This dedicated environment will help you engage more deeply in your Pilates practice, allowing you to fully reap the benefits of this fitness discipline.

Pilates Equipment and Accessories

When embarking on a Pilates practice, having the appropriate equipment and accessories is key to ensuring an effective and satisfying workout. While Pilates can be done with just your body, the use of specific equipment can greatly enrich the experience and allow for a greater variety of exercises. In this chapter, we will explore the essential equipment and accessories for Pilates practice and how they can enhance your training experience.

Pilates Mat: A high-quality Pilates mat is one of the fundamental components for practice. This mat should provide adequate support for your body during exercises, be thick enough to protect your joints from pressure, and have a non-slip surface to ensure stability during movements. Choose a mat that suits your personal needs and the type of exercises you intend to perform.

The Wall (Pareda): If you have access to a Wall (Pareda), you can use it to perform a variety of Pilates exercises that involve the wall. The Wall can be used to improve flexibility, stability, and strength. Ensure that it is securely anchored to the wall to ensure your safety during exercises.

Resistance Bands: Resistance bands are versatile tools that can be used to add resistance to Pilates exercises. They are lightweight, easy to carry, and allow you to vary the intensity of exercises according to your needs. Resistance bands can be used to train a wide range of muscle groups, helping to improve strength and flexibility.

Pilates Balls: Pilates balls are useful accessories for various exercises that involve stability and balance. Placing the ball under different parts of the body during exercises can increase the challenge and activate stabilizing muscles. Pilates balls are often used for abdominal and core toning exercises.

Cushions and Pads: Cushions and pads can be used to provide support or enhance comfort during exercises. For example, a cushion can be placed under the head or back to make supine exercises more comfortable. These accessories can be particularly helpful for those with back issues or other physical constraints.

Advanced Equipment: For those seeking a more advanced practice, there are other specific pieces of equipment such as the Pilates chair, Pilates barrel, and Pilates reformer. These pieces of equipment are often used in studio Pilates classes and offer a wide range of advanced exercises for those looking for a greater challenge.

It's important to note that not all accessories are necessary for all levels of Pilates practitioners. Beginners can start with a mat and, if desired, gradually add other accessories as they progress in their practice. The choice of equipment should be based on your individual needs, training goals, and level of experience.

Regardless of the equipment you choose, ensure that it is of high quality and safe to use. Before starting any new Pilates practice with equipment, it is advisable to consult with an experienced instructor to receive instructions and ensure that you are performing exercises safely and effectively.

In conclusion, the right equipment and accessories can greatly enhance your Pilates practice, offering you more options and challenges during exercises. However, the choice of equipment should be based on your individual needs and your level of experience. Choose accessories that enhance your practice and help you achieve your fitness goals safely and effectively.

Safety and Comfort

Safety and comfort are two fundamental aspects that you should carefully consider when embarking on a Pilates practice. These elements are essential to ensure that your workout experience is not only effective but also free from health risks or injuries. In this chapter, we will explore the importance of maintaining a safe and comfortable training environment while practising Pilates.

First and foremost, safety is an absolute priority. During Pilates exercises, it is essential to perform movements correctly to avoid injuries. Before starting a new workout routine or a specific exercise, it is advisable to consult with a qualified Pilates instructor. An experienced instructor can guide you on the correct execution techniques, helping you prevent incorrect or harmful movements for your body.

One of the fundamental principles of Pilates is control of movements. This principle implies that every movement should be executed deliberately and with control. Maintaining control of movements not only enhances the effectiveness of exercises but also reduces the risk of injuries. Avoid abrupt or overly rapid movements that could jeopardize your safety.

The correct use of Pilates equipment is another crucial aspect of safety. Ensure that the mat and accessories are in good condition and well-positioned to prevent falls or accidents. Regularly check your equipment to ensure it is in excellent condition and replace any damaged components.

A clutter-free environment is essential for safety. Before starting your Pilates session, make sure that the space around you is free from furniture or other objects that could pose a danger during exercises. This is particularly important when performing exercises that require wide movements or body rotations.

As for comfort, it is important to feel at ease during Pilates practice. Wear comfortable and breathable clothing that allows for maximum freedom of movement. Lightweight and breathable fabrics are ideal for avoiding overheating during exercises.

If you have back problems or other physical conditions, you may need cushions or pads to increase comfort during exercises. These accessories can be placed under the head, back, or other parts of the body to reduce pressure and prevent discomfort.

The temperature of the training environment should be comfortable. The body tends to cool down during Pilates practice, so make sure to wear layers of clothing that you can add or remove as needed. Maintaining an appropriate room temperature will help avoid overheating or excessive cooling during practice.

Having water present during training is essential to maintain good hydration levels. Ensure you have a water bottle within reach and drink regularly during your Pilates session.

In conclusion, safety and comfort are essential aspects of Pilates practice. Performing exercises correctly and maintaining a clutter-free environment are fundamental for safety. Wearing comfortable clothing and having access to water contribute to comfort during training. Take the time to create a training environment that is safe and enjoyable so that you can fully benefit from

Pilates without worrying about health risks or physical discomfort.

Creating an Effective Workout Routine

Creating an effective workout routine is an essential step to maximize the benefits of your Pilates practice. A well-structured routine helps you maintain consistency in your training, achieve your fitness goals, and fully utilize the principles of Pilates. In this chapter, we will explore how to create a personalized workout routine that suits your needs and goals.

The first step in creating a successful workout routine is to establish clear and realistic goals. Ask yourself what you want to achieve from your Pilates practice. Do you want to improve your flexibility, increase core strength, or reduce back pain? Once you've identified your goals, you can tailor your routine to focus on those specific aspects.

The frequency of your workouts is another important element to consider. Determine how many times a week you want to dedicate to Pilates. Many practitioners find it beneficial to work out at least three or four times a week to see tangible results. However, the frequency can vary based on your current fitness level and time availability.

After establishing your goals and frequency, you can start planning the structure of your workout routine. A basic Pilates routine often includes a variety of exercises that engage the core, upper and lower body, as well as flexibility exercises. You can break down your routine into sessions to focus on specific muscle groups or follow a more balanced approach that engages the entire body.

The duration of each workout session is important to consider. While beginners can start with shorter sessions, such as 30 minutes, experienced practitioners may dedicate up to 60-90 minutes for a complete practice. The key is to maintain the quality of the exercises rather than the quantity of time spent.

A crucial part of creating a successful workout routine is diversifying your exercises. Vary exercises and training modalities to prevent boredom and continuously challenge your body. Incorporate bodyweight Pilates exercises, the use of equipment like resistance bands or Pilates balls, and integrate the Wall (Pareda) if available.

Balancing strength and flexibility exercises is fundamental in Pilates. Make sure to include a combination of exercises that target core and limb strength, as well as exercises that improve flexibility and mobility. This will help create a strong and balanced body.

To keep your workout routine interesting and motivating, you can also consider using guided Pilates videos led by experienced instructors. These videos offer a variety and detailed instructions to help you perform exercises correctly.

Finally, consistency is crucial for achieving lasting results. Commit to following your workout routine regularly and over the long term. Monitor your progress and adjust your routine when necessary to continue reaching new goals.

In conclusion, creating a personalized workout routine is a crucial step to maximize the benefits of Pilates practice. Set clear goals, plan the frequency and duration of sessions, vary your exercises, and maintain consistency in your training. A well-structured routine will help you improve your strength, flexibility, and overall well-being, allowing you to fully enjoy the principles of Pilates and its lasting benefits.

Mindset and Awareness

Mindset and awareness are key elements in Pilates practice, influencing not only how you perform exercises but also how you approach your body and overall well-being. In this chapter, we will explore the importance of developing a positive mindset and body awareness in your Pilates practice.

Mindset is your mental attitude towards Pilates practice. It's essential to approach your training with an open, positive, and patient mindset. Pilates is a discipline that takes time to develop the strength, flexibility, and coordination required for advanced exercises. Embracing the learning process and not expecting immediate results is crucial.

A positive mindset can also help you overcome challenges and obstacles along the way. You may encounter exercises that seem difficult at first, but instead of becoming discouraged, view these challenges as opportunities to grow and improve. A positive mindset allows you to face challenges with determination and perseverance.

Body awareness is another fundamental aspect of Pilates. It means being aware of your body, its movements, and the sensations you experience during exercises. Body awareness helps you perform exercises more precisely and effectively. You can focus on how each part of your body moves and interacts during a specific exercise.

One of the keys to developing body awareness is concentration. During Pilates practice, you should fully concentrate on the exercise you're performing. Eliminate mental distractions and direct your attention to the movement. This concentration not only improves the quality of exercises but also promotes a sense of calm and mental well-being.

Breathing is another crucial aspect of body awareness. In Pilates, breathing is coordinated with movements. Learning to breathe in a controlled and rhythmic manner during exercises helps maintain balance, stability, and fluidity of movements. Controlled breathing also provides the necessary oxygen to the working muscles.

Body awareness helps you prevent overloading or overusing certain parts of the body. Often, in many fitness disciplines, we tend to overuse strong muscles and neglect weaker ones. Body awareness allows you to evenly distribute the work among muscles, helping maintain balance and preventing overload injuries.

An important aspect of body awareness is also postural correction. Pilates promotes proper posture and body alignment. Being aware of your posture and alignment during exercises helps you maintain good posture in your daily life, reducing the risk of back strains and pains.

In conclusion, developing a positive mindset and body awareness are essential elements in Pilates practice. These aspects enhance the quality of your exercises, promote mental and physical well-being, and help prevent injuries. Pilates is much more than just a physical workout; it's a holistic approach that connects mind and body, leading to increased awareness and lasting improvement in overall well-being. By working on your mindset and body awareness, you can fully reap the benefits of Pilates and enjoy a healthier and more harmonious life.

Chapter 4: "Basic Exercises to Strengthen Your Body with the Wall"

Introduction to Wall Exercises

The introduction to wall exercises represents a crucial step in your Pilates journey, as it allows you to discover how to use this versatile tool to enhance your body's strength, stability, and flexibility. The Wall, also known as "The Wall" or "The Wall Unit," is a fundamental component of Pilates that offers a range of unique benefits. In this chapter, we will explore the key concepts behind wall exercises and how they can enrich your practice.

The Wall is a special structure designed to support a wide range of Pilates exercises. It consists of a solid framework with horizontal and vertical bars, as well as attachments for straps and resistance bands. This tool provides a secure and stable support for performing a variety of whole-body exercises.

One of the primary advantages of wall exercises is the ability to harness the resistance of gravity in different ways. You can perform vertical, horizontal, and angled exercises, each with specific effects on your body. For example, vertical exercises can improve leg and lower-body strength, while horizontal ones can focus on core stability and posture.

Furthermore, the Wall provides support for improving flexibility. Stretching exercises with the Wall allows for greater extension and flexibility, as you can use the wall as an anchor point to safely and effectively stretch your muscles.

Another key aspect of wall exercises is the ability to work on joint mobility. The various positions and angling options allow you to engage different joints, helping to maintain their full range of motion and prevent stiffness.

The Wall is particularly beneficial for those looking to develop core strength. Many Pilates positions with the Wall significantly engage the core, helping you build a stable strength foundation. This is crucial for improving posture, preventing back pain, and achieving greater overall strength.

It is important to note that while the Wall offers numerous benefits, it is essential to use it safely and under the guidance of a qualified instructor, especially if you are new to Pilates. An experienced instructor will guide you in the proper execution of exercises, ensuring that you maintain the correct posture and alignment to prevent injuries.

The Wall can be an exciting and motivating addition to your Pilates practice, offering you new challenges and growth opportunities. During wall exercises, remember to focus on your breathing, body awareness, and the precision of movements. These aspects are crucial for getting the maximum benefits from each Wall workout session.

In conclusion, the introduction to wall exercises opens doors to a new dimension in your Pilates practice. This versatile tool provides unique opportunities to enhance body strength, stability, flexibility, and posture. Under the guidance of a qualified instructor, you can unlock the full potential of the Wall and how it can enrich your Pilates journey.

Exercise 1: Wall Squat

The "Wall Squat" exercise is a fundamental component in Pilates practice using the Wall as a support tool. This exercise aims to improve leg, glute, and core strength while promoting overall body stability and balance. When performed correctly, the "Wall Squat" can help develop a strong strength foundation and improve overall posture.

To perform the "Wall Squat," follow these steps:

Facing the Wall

1. Initial Position: Start by standing in front of the Wall. Ensure that the Wall is stable and securely anchored to the wall. Maintain a distance of about two steps from the Wall.

2. Body Alignment: Make sure to maintain good posture throughout the exercise. Your spine should be aligned, shoulders relaxed, and core engaged. Your feet should be slightly wider than shoulder-width apart, with toes pointing slightly outward.

3. Hand Position: Extend your arms forward, with your palms resting on the Wall at approximately shoulder height. Maintain a firm but not overly tight grip on the Wall.

4. Squat Movement: Begin to slowly bend your knees, lowering your body down as if you were about to sit on an imaginary chair. Keep your body weight evenly distributed on your heels and the balls of your feet. Continue to descend until your thighs are parallel to the floor or until you feel comfortable.

5. Chest Expansion: As you perform the squat movement, try to keep your chest open and your chest lifted. This helps

maintain proper posture and engages the core.

6. Breathing: Coordinate your breathing with the movement. Inhale as you begin to bend your knees and perform the downward movement. Exhale as you slowly return to an upright position. Controlled breathing helps stabilize the core during the exercise.

7. Controlled Execution: Perform the squat movement with control, avoiding jerky or overly fast motions. Focus on stability and balance throughout the exercise.

8. Repetitions: You can start with a moderate number of repetitions, such as 8-10, to get used to the exercise. As you gain confidence and strength, you can gradually increase the number of repetitions.

9. Progressive Strengthening: To increase the challenge, you can also use resistance bands or light weights while performing the "Wall Squat." These added accessories can help increase resistance and further develop muscle strength.

10. Safety: Ensure that you perform the exercise safely and under the supervision of a qualified instructor, especially if you

are new to Pilates or have specific physical conditions. Avoid pushing beyond your limits and always listen to your body.

In conclusion, the "Wall Squat" is an effective exercise for developing leg, glute, and core strength in Pilates practice. By following the correct instructions and focusing on posture and breathing, you can derive maximum benefits from this exercise. Gradually incorporate the "Wall Squat" into your Pilates routine to improve your overall strength and stability.

Exercise 2: Wall Push-Up

The "Wall Push-Up" exercise is a significant element in Pilates practice as it allows you to strengthen the chest, shoulders, triceps, and core while utilizing the Wall as a support tool. When performed correctly, this exercise can significantly improve upper body strength and overall stability. In this section, we will explore how to perform the "Wall Push-Up" effectively and its benefits for your body.

1. Initial Position: Start by standing facing the Wall, at a distance of about two steps. Ensure that the Wall is stable and securely anchored to the wall. Maintain

an upright posture with the spine aligned, shoulders relaxed, and core engaged.

2. Hand Position: Extend both arms forward and place the palms of your hands on the Wall, positioning them approximately shoulder-width apart. Your hands should be slightly wider than shoulder-width, with fingers pointing upwards.

3. Push-Up Movement: Inhale as you slowly bend your elbows, lowering your body towards the Wall. Keep your body aligned from head to toe, avoiding tilting your pelvis or sticking out your buttocks. Continue to descend until your chest is close to the Wall or until you feel comfortable.

4. Chest Expansion: During the push-up movement, try to keep your chest open and your chest lifted. This helps effectively engage the chest and shoulder muscles.

5. Breathing: Coordinate your breathing with the movement. Exhale as you push your body back up to the initial position. Inhale as you bend your elbows again to perform the next push-up.

6. Controlled Execution: Perform the push-up movement in a controlled manner,

avoiding abrupt or too fast motions. Focus on stability and strength during the exercise.

7. Repetitions: You can start with a moderate number of repetitions, such as 8-10, to get accustomed to the exercise. Over time, you can gradually increase the number of repetitions to increase the challenge.

8. Variations: To vary the intensity of the exercise, you can adjust the position of your hands on the Wall. Higher positions make the exercise easier, while lower positions make it more challenging.

9. Progressive Strengthening: If you desire further challenges, you can use resistance bands or light weights during the exercise to increase resistance.

10. Safety: Ensure that you perform the exercise safely and under the supervision of a qualified instructor, especially if you are new to Pilates or have specific physical conditions. Respect your limits and always listen to your body to avoid injuries.

In conclusion, the "Wall Push-Up" is an effective exercise to strengthen the upper body, including the chest, shoulders, and triceps. When performed correctly, this exercise will help develop a solid strength foundation and improve overall stability. Integrating the "Wall Push-Up" into your Pilates routine can lead to significant improvements in upper body strength and tone, contributing to your overall well-being.

Exercise 3: Wall Plank

The "Wall Plank" exercise is an important component in Pilates practice that utilizes the Wall as a support tool. This exercise aims to improve core stability, and arm and shoulder strength, and promote good posture and better body awareness. When performed with precision, the "Wall Plank" can significantly contribute to your overall well-being.

1. Initial Position: To begin the exercise, position yourself facing the Wall, maintaining a distance of about one step from it. Ensure that the Wall is stable and securely anchored to the wall. Maintain an upright posture with the spine aligned, shoulders relaxed, and the core engaged.

2. Hand Position: Extend both arms forward and place the palms of your hands on the Wall, positioning them at shoulder height. Your hands should be slightly wider than

shoulder-width, with fingers pointing upward.

3. Plank Movement: Inhale as you bend your elbows and bring your body closer to the Wall, keeping your body aligned from head to feet. The arms should be bent at an angle of approximately 90 degrees. Keep the core engaged and the pelvis aligned with the spine.

4. Stability and Breathing: During the exercise, focus on core stability. Maintain regular and controlled breathing. Exhale as you hold the position, keeping your body in a straight line. Inhale while slightly relaxing without allowing your body to sag.

5. Controlled Execution: Perform the "Wall Plank" in a controlled manner, avoiding pushing beyond your limits or collapsing in the pelvis. Concentrate on stability and strength throughout the exercise.

6. Holding Time: You can start with a moderate holding time, such as 20-30 seconds, to get accustomed to the exercise. As you gain strength and endurance, you can gradually increase the holding time to one minute or more.

7. Variations: To vary the intensity of the exercise, you can adjust the distance between you and the Wall. Greater distance increases the challenge. Additionally, you can perform the "Wall Plank" with one arm or one raised leg to increase the difficulty.

8. Safety: Ensure that you perform the exercise safely and under the supervision of a qualified instructor, especially if you are new to Pilates or have specific physical conditions. Respect your limits and listen to your body to avoid injuries.

In conclusion, the "Wall Plank" is a highly effective exercise for improving core stability, and arm and shoulder strength, and promoting correct posture. When performed with precision and gradual progression, this exercise can lead to significant benefits for your body. Integrating the "Wall Plank" into your Pilates routine will help improve your core strength, overall stability, and body awareness, thus supporting your overall well-being.

Exercise 4: Wall Stretching

The "Wall Stretching" exercise is a fundamental component in Pilates practice that uses the Wall as a support tool to improve flexibility, joint mobility, and muscle relaxation. This type of exercise allows you to leverage the stability of the Wall to safely and effectively perform a series of stretches targeting different muscle groups. When performed correctly, "Wall Stretching" can help prevent muscle tension, improve posture, and promote an overall sense of relaxation and well-being.

Initial Position: To begin, position yourself facing the Wall, maintaining a distance of one or two steps from it. Ensure that the Wall is stable and securely anchored to the wall. Maintain an upright posture with the spine aligned, shoulders relaxed, and the core engaged.

Hamstring Stretch: To stretch the hamstrings, place one foot on the Wall, keeping the leg slightly bent. Lean your torso forward with a straight back, and try to reach the foot placed on the Wall. You will feel a pleasant stretch along the back of the leg.

Calf Muscle Stretch: To stretch the calf muscles, position the right foot forward and the left foot backwards, keeping the left heel in contact with the floor and the leg extended. Place both hands on the Wall and push your hips slightly forward, feeling the relaxation of the calf muscles.

Lower Back and Lumbar Stretch: To stretch the lower back and lumbar region, place both hands on the Wall and walk backwards with your feet until your body is leaning forward and your back is straight. Maintain this position, allowing your body to relax and stretch in the lumbar area.

Shoulder and Chest Stretch: To stretch the shoulders and chest, place both hands on the Wall slightly higher than shoulder height. Gradually walk backwards with your feet while keeping your arms extended, allowing your chest to open up and your shoulders to stretch.

Arm and Bicep Stretch: To stretch the arms and biceps, place both hands on the Wall at shoulder height or slightly higher. Keep your arms extended and slowly lean your body forward, feeling the relaxation of the arm muscles.

Breathing and Relaxation: During each Wall Stretching exercise, focus on deep and controlled breathing. Inhale slowly through the nose and exhale through the mouth as you relax into the various stretches. This helps promote muscle relaxation and body awareness.

Safety and Gradual Progression: Perform all Wall Stretching exercises with care and gradual progression, avoiding excessive muscle strain. Always listen to your body and stop the exercise if you experience pain or discomfort.

Long-Lasting Benefits: Integrating "Wall Stretching" into your Pilates routine can lead to increased flexibility, improved joint mobility, and overall body relaxation. These benefits can help improve your posture, prevent muscle tension, and promote a sense of well-being.

In conclusion, "Wall Stretching" is an effective way to enhance flexibility, joint mobility, and muscle relaxation in Pilates practice. When performed correctly and gradually, this type of stretching can lead to lasting benefits for your body. Add "Wall Stretching" to your Pilates routine to enhance your physical and mental well-being.

Chapter 5: "In-Depth: Advanced Exercises to Challenge Your Strength"

Introduction to Advanced Exercises

The introduction to advanced exercises marks a milestone in your Pilates practice. After building a solid foundation of knowledge and strength with basic exercises, it's time to push yourself further and challenge your body in new and stimulating ways. Advanced exercises offer the opportunity to test your strength, flexibility, and endurance on a deeper level, taking the benefits of Pilates to the next level.

When you begin exploring advanced exercises, it's important to do so with care and awareness. These movements require greater technical precision and a deeper understanding of Pilates principles. They are designed to engage not only the superficial muscles but also the deep ones, helping to develop balanced strength and greater body awareness.

One of the primary goals of advanced exercises is gradual progression. Before attempting advanced exercises, it's essential to have a solid foundation of strength and a good grasp of Pilates' basic techniques. This will ensure that you are ready to tackle more complex challenges safely and effectively.

Among the advanced exercises we will explore in this chapter are the Suspended Plank with the Wall Unit, the Inverted Roll-Up with the Wall Unit, the Leg Circle with the Wall Unit, and the Swan Dive with the Wall Unit. Each of these exercises requires a combination of strength, flexibility, and core control, offering a variety of benefits, including muscle strengthening, improved posture, and enhanced balance.

During the execution of advanced exercises, proper breathing plays a crucial role. Synchronizing your breath with movement helps maintain stability and control while allowing your muscles to work optimally. Learning to breathe mindfully and in a controlled manner while tackling these challenges will be essential.

It's important to remember that Pilates practice is highly individualized. This means that your body may respond differently than someone else's to advanced exercises. Therefore, it's crucial to always listen to your body and respect your limits. Don't try to force movements or take big steps too soon. Gradual progression and respecting your personal limits are key to reaping the maximum benefits of advanced exercises without risking injury.

Throughout this chapter, we will provide detailed instructions on the correct technique and breathing for each of the advanced exercises. This guide will help you fully understand how to perform these complex movements safely and effectively, allowing you to deepen your Pilates practice and make the most of the benefits it offers. It will be a challenge, but also an opportunity to discover new dimensions of your physical strength and body awareness.

Exercise 1: Suspended Plank with the Wall Unit

The "Suspended Plank with the Wall Unit" exercise is one of the pillars of advanced Pilates exercises that demands significant core, arm, and shoulder strength. This advanced variation of the standard plank involves using the Wall Unit as an anchoring point for your hands, creating a suspended position that increases the challenge and requires more control and strength to maintain balance and stability. In this section, we will explore in detail how to correctly perform the "Suspended Plank with the Wall Unit" to derive maximum benefit from your practice.

Initial Positioning: Begin by positioning yourself in front of the Wall Unit, at a distance of about one step from it. Ensure that the Wall Unit is securely anchored to the wall and stable. Maintain an upright posture with a straight spine, relaxed shoulders, and an engaged core.

Hand Position: Extend both arms forward and place the palms of your hands on the Wall Unit, positioning them at shoulder height. Your hands should be slightly wider than shoulder-width apart, with your fingers pointing upward. Ensure that your hands are securely anchored to the Wall Unit to support your weight.

Suspended Plank Movement: Inhale slowly, bend your elbows, and lean your body forward, pushing your hips upward and lifting your feet off the floor, creating a suspended position. Keep your body aligned from head to toe, avoiding tilting your hips or sticking out your buttocks.

Control and Stability: Focus on stability and control as you maintain the suspended position. Your core should be engaged to the maximum, and you should feel significant tension in the abdominal, arm, and shoulder muscles. Maintain regular and deep breathing to sustain your effort.

Chest Expansion: During the "Suspended Plank with the Wall Unit," aim to keep your chest open and your chest lifted. This helps engage the shoulder muscles and maintain proper posture.

Suspension Time: You can start with a moderate suspension time, such as 15-20 seconds, to get accustomed to the exercise. As you gain strength and endurance, you can gradually increase the suspension time to one minute or more.

Advanced Variation: To further increase the challenge, you can lift one leg off the Wall Unit during the "Suspended Plank," alternating between legs. This requires additional core and trunk strength.

Safety: It's essential to perform this exercise safely and under the supervision of a qualified instructor, especially if you are new to advanced Pilates exercises. Always respect your limits and listen to your body to avoid injuries.

In conclusion, the "Suspended Plank with the Wall Unit" is an advanced exercise that tests your core, arm, and shoulder strength, also requiring significant control and stability. When executed correctly, this exercise can lead to significant improvements in overall body strength and tone. By incorporating it into your advanced Pilates practice, you can fully harness the benefits of this challenging exercise to enhance your overall well-being.

Exercise 2: Inverted Roll-Up with the Wall Unit

The "Inverted Roll-Up with the Wall Unit" exercise is an advanced Pilates variation that challenges spinal flexibility, core strength, and coordination. This complex movement requires a good understanding of basic Pilates techniques and mastery of previous exercises. Let's explore in detail how to correctly perform the "Inverted Roll-Up with the Wall Unit" to derive maximum benefit from your advanced practice.

Initial Positioning: To begin, sit on the floor facing the Wall Unit, with your legs extended and your body lengthened. Ensure that the Wall Unit is stable and securely anchored to the wall. Maintain an upright posture with a straight spine, relaxed shoulders, and an engaged core.

Hand Position: Extend both arms forward and grasp the Wall Unit with your hands, positioning them slightly wider than shoulder-width apart. Your hands should be facing the ceiling. This will be your grip during the exercise.

Inverted Roll-Up Movement: Inhale slowly, bend your body forward from the waist, tilting your pelvis and rolling your spine toward the floor. Keep your legs extended, and aim to reach the floor with the upper part of your back as you roll down.

Control and Coordination: The "Inverted Roll-Up with the Wall Unit" requires significant coordination and control. During the movement, try to keep your core engaged and control the movement of your spine. Your goal is to roll down slowly and in a controlled manner toward the floor.

Arrival in the Vertical Position: Continue rolling slowly until you reach the vertical position, with your body fully aligned. Maintain this position for a moment, allowing the core and back muscles to work stabilizing.

Return to the Starting Position: Exhale as you begin to unroll your spine slowly, starting from the upper back, until you return to the initial seated position while maintaining control of the movement.

Repetitions and Breathing: Start with a limited number of repetitions, such as 3-5, to get accustomed to the exercise. Maintain regular breathing throughout the movement, inhaling as you roll down and exhaling as you return to the seated position.

Safety: Safe execution of the exercise is of paramount importance, especially when dealing with complex movements like the "Inverted Roll-Up with the Wall Unit." Ensure that you perform it under the supervision of a qualified instructor, especially if you are new to advanced Pilates exercises.

Benefits: This advanced exercise is designed to improve spinal flexibility, core strength, and coordination. It's an excellent way to challenge your skills and take your Pilates practice to a new level. Beyond the physical benefits, the controlled execution of the "Inverted Roll-Up with the Wall Unit" requires mental concentration, promoting body awareness.

In conclusion, the "Inverted Roll-Up with the Wall Unit" is an advanced exercise that presents a stimulating challenge for your body and mind. When executed with correct technique and adequate control, it can lead to significant improvements in spinal flexibility, core strength, and coordination. Integrating this exercise into your advanced Pilates practice can provide a rewarding experience and promote your overall well-being.

Exercise 3: Leg Circle with the Wall Unit

The "Leg Circle with the Wall Unit" exercise is an advanced Pilates movement that focuses on leg strength, flexibility, and core stability. This exercise is a challenging variation of the classic "Leg Circles" and utilizes the Wall Unit as an anchoring point to provide increased resistance and an added challenge to the leg and core muscles. In the following description, we will explore in detail how to correctly perform the "Leg Circle with the Wall Unit" to reap the maximum benefits from your advanced Pilates practice.

Initial Positioning: Start by sitting on the floor, facing the Wall Unit, with your legs extended and your body elongated. Ensure that the Wall Unit is stable and securely anchored to the wall. Maintain an upright posture with a straight spine, relaxed shoulders, and an engaged core.

Hand Position: Grip the Wall Unit with both hands, positioning them slightly wider than shoulder-width apart. Your hands should be securely anchored to the Wall Unit as this will be your grip during the exercise.

Leg Circle Movement: Inhale as you lift one leg off the floor and raise it upward toward the ceiling. Keep the leg extended and the foot flexed. From here, start drawing circles with the leg, moving it in a clockwise or counterclockwise direction. Try to maintain control of the movement and avoid excessive swinging.

Control and Coordination: The "Leg Circle with the Wall Unit" requires significant coordination between the legs and the core. The core should be engaged to stabilize the lower body as the legs execute controlled circles. Maintain regular breathing throughout the movement, inhaling as the leg ascends and exhaling as it descends.

Repetitions and Leg Switch: Perform a limited number of repetitions, such as 5-8 circles in a clockwise direction and 5-8 circles in a counterclockwise direction with one leg before switching to the other. Keep the leg movement controlled and precise.

Advanced Variation: To increase the challenge, you can perform the "Leg Circle with the Wall Unit" with the raised leg positioned higher or with wider circle diameters. This requires greater leg and core strength.

Safety: Ensure that you perform this exercise safely and under the supervision of a qualified instructor, especially if you are new to advanced Pilates exercises. Respect your limits and listen to your body to avoid injuries.

Benefits: The "Leg Circle with the Wall Unit" is an advanced exercise that focuses on leg strength, flexibility, and core control. This movement is excellent for developing greater awareness of the legs and improving lower body strength. Additionally, it helps strengthen the stabilizing muscles of the core, promoting better posture and increased trunk stability.

In conclusion, the "Leg Circle with the Wall Unit" is an advanced exercise that offers a stimulating challenge for the legs, core, and coordination. When performed with correct technique and control, it can lead to significant improvements in leg and core strength and stability. Integrating this exercise into your advanced Pilates practice can contribute to strengthening your body and enhancing your overall body awareness.

Exercise 4: Swan Dive with the Wall Unit

The "Swan Dive with the Wall Unit" exercise is an advanced variation in Pilates aimed at improving spinal flexibility, core strength, and upper body mobility. This complex movement engages various muscle groups and requires precise coordination. In the following description, we will explore in detail how to correctly perform the "Swan Dive with the Wall Unit" to reap the maximum benefits from your advanced Pilates practice.

Initial Positioning: Begin by sitting on the floor, facing the Wall Unit, with your legs extended and your body elongated. Ensure that the Wall Unit is securely anchored to the wall and stable. Maintain an upright posture with a straight spine, relaxed shoulders, and an engaged core.

Hand Position: Extend both arms forward and grip the Wall Unit with your hands, positioning them slightly wider than shoulder-width apart. Your hands should be facing the ceiling. This will be your grip during the exercise.

Swan Dive Movement: Inhale as you begin to lift your torso slowly from the waist, lengthening the spine upward. Imagine bending forward from the chest, as if you were trying to reach the ceiling with your chest. Keep your legs and feet on the ground.

Back Extension: Continue lifting the torso, elongating the spine in a fluid motion. Try to keep the shoulders relaxed and open, and imagine lengthening the neck to avoid tension.

Control and Stability: The "Swan Dive with the Wall Unit" requires significant control and stability. Engage your core to support the movement of the spine, and the muscles of the back should work in coordination. Maintain regular breathing throughout the movement, inhaling as you lift the torso and exhaling as you return to the seated position.

Arrival in the Extended Position: When you have lifted the torso enough, reach maximum extension, aiming to create a straight line between your head and hips. Hold this position for a moment to fully benefit from the spine's elongation.

Return to the Starting Position: Exhale as you begin to slowly bend the torso downward from the waist, returning to the initial seated position. Try to maintain control of the movement during this return phase.

Repetitions and Breathing: Start with a limited number of repetitions, such as 3-5, to get accustomed to the exercise. Maintain regular breathing throughout the movement, following your body's rhythm.

Safety: Safe execution of the exercise is of utmost importance, especially when dealing with complex movements like the "Swan Dive with the Wall Unit." Make sure to perform it under the supervision of a qualified instructor, especially if you are new to advanced Pilates exercises. Always respect your limits and listen to your body to prevent injuries.

Benefits: The "Swan Dive with the Wall Unit" is an advanced exercise that offers a stimulating challenge for spinal flexibility, core strength, and upper body mobility. This movement is ideal for improving posture, strengthening trunk muscles, and promoting better overall flexibility and mobility. In addition to physical benefits, it requires mental concentration, promoting body awareness.

In conclusion, the "Swan Dive with the Wall Unit" is an advanced exercise that represents a stimulating challenge for your flexibility, core strength, and spinal mobility. When performed with correct technique and control, it can lead to significant improvements in posture and trunk strength. Integrating this exercise into your advanced Pilates practice can contribute to strengthening your body and enhancing your overall body awareness.

Chapter 6: Continuous Flow: Creating a Pilates Wall Unit Workout Routine

Structuring Your Routine

Structuring your Pilates wall unit workout routine is crucial to maximize benefits and ensure effective practice. a well-organized routine will help you maintain a continuous flow, work on different muscle groups, and achieve measurable results over time. In this chapter, we will explore how to structure your routine to maximize your time and effort during your workout.

1. Defining Goals: Before you start structuring your routine, it's important to have clear goals for your Pilates wall unit training. Do you want to improve your strength? Increase flexibility? Enhance your posture? Knowing your goals will help you select the most appropriate exercises and plan the duration of your session.

2. Exercise Selection: Once you've defined your goals, you can choose the exercises that will help you achieve them. For example, if your goal is to increase core strength, you can include exercises like "Suspended Plank with the Wall Unit" and

"Leg Circle with the Wall Unit." If you're working on flexibility, you might focus on exercises that involve controlled, expansive movements.

3. Exercise Order: The order of exercises is important to maintain flow during your routine. Begin with light warm-up exercises to prepare your body, then progress to more challenging ones. For instance, you could start with a set of "Squats with the Wall Unit" to warm up your legs and core, then move on to exercises like the "Swan Dive with the Wall Unit" to work on spinal flexibility.

4. Routine Duration: The duration of your routine depends on your goals and fitness level. In general, a Pilates wall unit workout routine can range from 20 minutes to an hour or more. It's essential to balance the duration with exercise intensity and your personal capacity. Start with a reasonable duration and gradually increase it as you gain strength and endurance.

5. Progression: Progression is crucial for achieving long-term results. Gradually increase the intensity of exercises and add more advanced variations as your body adapts. Progression prevents

stagnation and keeps your routine interesting and challenging.

6. Listening to Your Body: Finally, it's essential to listen to your body during your routine. If you feel pain or excessive tension, stop and modify the exercise or position. Safety is paramount, so avoid pushing your body beyond its limits.

Overall, structuring your Pilates wall unit workout routine will help you maximize benefits and maintain a continuous flow during your practice. A well-planned routine will allow you to effectively reach your goals, contributing to your physical and mental well-being.

Effective Sequences

Effective sequences play a crucial role in your Pilates wall unit workout routine. A well-structured sequence allows for a continuous flow during practice, engages various muscle groups, and leads to measurable results over time. In this chapter, we'll delve into the importance of effective sequences and how you can create a series of exercises that integrate smoothly and harmoniously.

1. Continuous Flow: One of the keys to an effective sequence is a continuous flow.

Exercises should naturally connect, enabling a seamless transition from one movement to the next. This flow keeps the energy high during the session and makes the workout more engaging.

2. Muscular Balance: Sequences should be designed to involve a balance of muscle groups. For instance, after an exercise that engages the core and legs, you might transition to one that targets the upper body or focuses on spinal flexibility. This balance contributes to developing a harmonious and well-rounded body.

3. Progression: Progression is a key element of effective sequences. Start with warm-up exercises and gradually increase intensity and complexity as you progress through the sequence. This allows your body to adapt progressively to the training and achieve lasting results.

4. Variation: Effective sequences include intelligent variation in exercises. Changing the angle, hand position, or movements can provide a new challenge to your muscles and prevent monotony. Variation can also prevent the development of muscle resistance to constant overload.

5. Coordinated Breathing: Coordinating breathing with movements is essential for an effective sequence. Deep and controlled breathing helps maintain stability and concentration during the workout. Be sure to follow the breathing cues for each exercise.

6. Flexibility and Mobility: Sequences should include exercises that work on flexibility and joint mobility. These movements can prevent muscle tension and improve the range of motion. For example, you can incorporate stretching or chest-opening exercises within the sequence.

7. Adaptability: An effective sequence is adaptable to your individual needs. You can adjust the sequence based on your fitness level, specific goals, and any physical limitations. This flexibility allows you to derive the maximum benefit from your training.

8. Listening to Your Body: Finally, during the sequence, it's crucial to listen closely to your body. If you experience pain or excessive tension, it's essential to stop and, if necessary, modify the exercise or position. Your safety always comes first.

In conclusion, effective sequences are essential to maximize the benefits of your Pilates wall unit workout routine. A well-structured sequence maintains a continuous flow, engages a variety of muscle groups, and adapts to your individual needs. When you create thoughtful and balanced sequences, you increase the likelihood of achieving positive results in your Pilates practice.

Flexibility and Adaptability

Flexibility and adaptability are key concepts when it comes to structuring a Pilates wall unit workout routine. These two elements are crucial to ensure that your practice is effective, safe, and tailored to your individual needs.

Flexibility in Routine Design:

Flexibility in routine design means being able to adapt your Pilates workout to address a variety of goals and fitness levels. This is particularly important because each individual has different objectives when it comes to Pilates. Some people may be seeking to improve core strength, while others may focus on spinal flexibility or posture correction. A well-structured routine should be flexible enough to allow each individual to pursue their specific goals.

Furthermore, flexibility in routine design allows you to customize your Pilates workout to accommodate any physical limitations or medical conditions. For example, if you have a back issue, you can tailor your routine to avoid exercises that might exert pressure on the lumbar area.

Adaptability to Progression:

Adaptability is also crucial when it comes to the progression of your Pilates practice. Pilates is a discipline that aims for gradual progression. As your body adapts to the exercises, it's essential to gradually introduce more challenging variations to continue challenging yourself.

An experienced Pilates instructor will be able to adapt your routine based on your fitness level and specific needs. For example, you might start with basic exercises to build a strong foundation and then progress to more advanced exercises as you gain strength, balance, and flexibility. Adaptability to progression is crucial to avoid stagnation and achieve lasting results.

Flexibility during Exercise Execution:

Flexibility doesn't just apply to routine design; it also pertains to your ability to adapt during exercise execution. During a Pilates session, you may find that on some days you feel more flexible and able to perform an exercise with a wider range of motion, while on other days, you may experience more tension or stiffness. It's important to listen to your body and adjust the intensity and range of motion based on how you feel at the moment.

Adaptability during exercise execution is a key component of safety. If you feel pain or excessive tension, it's important to immediately modify the exercise or position to prevent injuries. Your Pilates practice should be challenging but also a safe and comfortable experience.

In conclusion, flexibility and adaptability are two essential aspects of creating and executing a Pilates wall unit workout routine. Flexibility in routine design allows you to personalize your training to fit your goals and needs. Adaptability to progression helps you grow gradually in your Pilates journey. Moreover, flexibility during exercise execution ensures a safe and comfortable practice. Whether you're a beginner starting your Pilates journey or an experienced practitioner, these principles remain fundamental for a successful and rewarding practice.

Breathing and Flow

Breathing and flow are interconnected fundamental elements in Pilates wall unit training. Coordinated breathing with movements is a distinctive aspect of this discipline, contributing to creating a continuous flow and enhancing the effectiveness of the workout. In this chapter, we will explore how breathing and flow work together to create a comprehensive and rewarding Pilates practice.

Breathing as a Guide:

In Pilates, breathing is more than just a physiological function; it is an essential tool for guiding movements and flow. During exercises, breathing is synchronized with movements precisely. Typically, diaphragmatic breathing is used, involving the diaphragm to inhale and exhale slowly and in a controlled manner.

Breathing serves to stabilize the core, improve concentration, and prevent premature fatigue. When performing exercises that engage the core, such as "Plank with the Wall Unit," deep breathing helps maintain balance and stability during execution.

Synchronization with Flow:

Flow is what makes Pilates with the wall unit unique. Exercises are designed to flow seamlessly from one to another, creating a sequence of harmonious movements. Breathing plays a key role in this process as each inhalation and exhalation is synchronized with the movement.

For example, in an exercise like "Roll-Up with the Wall Unit," you inhale as you lift your torso and exhale as you gradually lower yourself to the mat. This respiratory synchronization helps maintain the rhythm and flow of the practice, contributing to the sense of continuity and fluidity.

Focus on Concentration:

Breathing and flow are not only physical aspects but also mental ones. Concentration is crucial in Pilates, and breathing is a tool to enhance your body awareness. When you focus on your breath, you become more present in the execution of exercises.

Breathing becomes a form of meditation in motion, helping you clear your mind from external distractions and connect with your body. This mindful approach improves your ability to control movements and perform exercises precisely and effectively.

Breathing for Comfort and Safety:

Proper breathing in Pilates also contributes to comfort and safety during training. Diaphragmatic breathing promotes the relaxation of superficial muscles and reduces tension. This is particularly useful when tackling challenging exercises, as it helps avoid muscle overload and prevents injuries.

Furthermore, synchronizing breathing with movement helps maintain sustainable flow. By breathing in a controlled manner, you can avoid fatigue and sustain a longer and more satisfying practice.

In conclusion, breathing and flow are two interconnected elements that make Pilates with the wall unit a unique and effective experience. Breathing guides movements, synchronizes flow, and enhances mental concentration. These aspects contribute to creating a comprehensive and rewarding practice that improves strength, flexibility, and body awareness. By integrating mindful breathing into your practice, you can derive the maximum benefit from Pilates wall unit training, enhancing your physical and mental well-being.

Maintaining Awareness

Maintaining awareness is a vital aspect of your Pilates wall unit training. Body awareness is the ability to be present in the moment, listen to your body, and understand how each movement affects your physiology. In this chapter, we will explore how to maintain awareness during your workout routine to maximize the benefits of Pilates.

1. Listening to Your Body:

One of the key elements of awareness is careful listening to your body. This means being able to identify physical sensations, muscle tensions, and the signals your body is sending you during exercise. When you are aware, you can promptly detect any signs of discomfort or tension and adjust your movement accordingly to prevent injuries.

2. Focus on the Movement:

Maintaining focus on the movement is another essential aspect of awareness. When you concentrate attentively on how you perform an exercise, you can ensure that each movement is precise and controlled. This attention to detail enhances the effectiveness of the exercise and helps prevent incorrect behaviours or abrupt movements that could lead to injuries.

3. Mindful Breathing:

Breathing is a crucial bridge between the body and mind in Pilates practice. Mindful breathing is the precise coordination of your inhalation and exhalation with movements. When you breathe in a controlled manner, you can improve the stability of your core and your mental concentration. Breath awareness also helps you maintain a continuous flow during the practice.

4. Knowing Your Limits and Abilities:

Awareness allows you to recognize your physical limits and current capabilities. This knowledge is crucial for safe and effective practice. For example, if you are new to Pilates, you should be aware of your limits and start with basic exercises. With experience, you can gradually expand your practice and challenge yourself more and more.

5. Mindfulness and Stress Reduction:

Maintaining awareness during Pilates can have benefits beyond the physical realm. The practice of mindfulness, which is intrinsic to mindful Pilates, can help reduce stress and anxiety. When you are immersed in your workout and set aside external distractions, you can experience a sense of calm and mental well-being.

6. Personal Growth and Self-Esteem:

Finally, awareness can contribute to personal growth and self-esteem. Every progress you make in your Pilates practice is a result of your dedication and your ability to listen to and understand your body. These successes can have a positive impact on your self-esteem and confidence in your abilities.

In conclusion, maintaining awareness is crucial in Pilates wall unit training. Body awareness helps you avoid injuries, perform exercises with precision, and fully reap the benefits of training. Furthermore, the mindfulness incorporated into your practice can enhance your mental well-being and self-esteem. Awareness is not only a physical component but also a mental and spiritual experience that can enrich your life in many ways.

Chapter 7: "Focus on Flexibility: Incorporating Stretching into Your Workouts"

The Importance of Stretching

The importance of stretching is a key element in your Pilates with Pareda practice. This chapter focuses on how improving flexibility contributes to your physical and mental well-being. Stretching is not just a pleasant addition to your workout routine, but it is essential for long-term success in Pilates and your overall health.

Improved Flexibility:

Stretching is the primary means of improving your muscle and joint flexibility. In the practice of Pilates with Pareda, flexibility is essential because many exercises require a full range of motion. A more flexible body allows you to perform exercises with greater precision and effectiveness while avoiding muscle tension or injuries.

Injury Prevention:

One of the primary benefits of stretching is injury prevention. A more flexible body is less susceptible to muscle strains, tears, and joint injuries. This is particularly important in Pilates with Pareda because exercises often involve the core, spine, and joints. Proper stretching prepares your body for challenging movements, reducing the risk of injuries.

Improved Posture:

Flexibility is closely related to good posture. One of the main goals of Pilates is to improve posture and postural awareness. Regular stretching of muscles that influence posture, such as those in the neck, shoulders, and back, can help you maintain an upright and balanced posture.

Relaxation and Stress Reduction:

Stretching also has a positive impact on your mind. Stretching exercises can promote muscle relaxation and reduce bodily tension. This relaxing effect can help reduce stress and anxiety, improving your overall sense of well-being. In Pilates with Pareda, the combination of stretching and controlled breathing promotes a sense of calm and mindfulness.

Performance Enhancement:

Increased flexibility can also enhance your performance in Pilates. When muscles are flexible, you can perform exercises more smoothly and precisely. This can lead to greater strength, stability, and control in your movements. Furthermore, flexibility can make it easier to perform advanced exercises.

Long-Term Results:

Stretching is a long-term investment in your physical health. Unlike temporary gains you might achieve with strength exercises, the flexibility gained through stretching persists over time. This means that you will be able to continue improving your flexibility and preventing injuries over the years.

In conclusion, the importance of stretching in Pilates with Pareda cannot be underestimated. It contributes to improved flexibility, injury prevention, maintaining good posture, reducing stress, and enhancing performance. Incorporating stretching exercises regularly into your practice will help you achieve longer-lasting results and keep your body in great shape.

Types of Stretching

In the context of Pilates with Pareda, there are several types of stretching that can be incorporated into your routine to improve flexibility and gain maximum benefits from your practice. These various types of stretching include static, dynamic, and assisted stretching, each with its specific purpose and application.

1. Static Stretching:

Static stretching is the most common and well-known type. It involves holding a stretched position for an extended period, typically ranging from 15 to 60 seconds. During static stretching, the muscle is taken to an elongated position and held there without movement. This type of stretching is useful for increasing muscle flexibility and improving the range of motion. Examples of static stretching in Pilates may include leg stretches or upper body stretches.

2. Dynamic Stretching:

Unlike static stretching, dynamic stretching involves controlled movement during stretching. Instead of holding a position, you perform continuous movements that engage a range of muscles and joints. This type of stretching can help improve functional flexibility and prepare the body for dynamic movements during Pilates practice. For example, performing leg swings before a leg exercise can be considered dynamic stretching.

3. Assisted Stretching:

Assisted stretching involves the use of a partner or special equipment to aid in stretching. This type of stretching is useful for achieving greater depth in stretching and focusing on specific areas of the body. In Pilates with Pareda, some equipment like resistance bands or pulleys can be used to provide assisted traction, allowing for deeper and targeted stretching.

4. Ballistic Stretching:

Ballistic stretching involves bouncing or swinging movements to increase muscle stretching. However, this type of stretching is often discouraged in Pilates, as it can increase the risk of injury or muscle strains. Pilates emphasizes movement control and precision, and ballistic stretching can interfere with these principles.

5. Proprioceptive Neuromuscular Facilitation (PNF) Stretching:

PNF stretching is a technique where the muscle to be stretched is contracted for a brief period before being stretched. This type of stretching can promote deeper muscle relaxation and improve flexibility. In Pilates, it's important to perform this type of stretching with care, focusing on the proper execution of movements.

The choice of which type of stretching to use will depend on the specific goals of your Pilates with Pareda practice and your personal preferences. It's important to note that Pilates emphasizes control, precision, and respect for the body's limits. So, any type of stretching you incorporate into your routine should be done mindfully and in line with Pilates principles. Always consult with a qualified instructor if you're unsure which type of stretching is appropriate for you or if you want specific guidance on proper technique.

Stretching Integration

Integrating stretching is an essential element in maximizing the benefits of your Pilates with Pareda practice. Stretching should not be considered as a separate addition to your routine but rather as an integral part of the training process. In this chapter, we will explore how you can effectively integrate stretching into your Pilates practice to achieve better results and maintain a healthy and flexible body.

1. Pre-Workout Preparation:

Before starting your Pilates with Pareda session, it's essential to prepare your body through stretching. This type of stretching should be dynamic and aimed at warming up the muscles and joints that will be engaged during the workout. Examples of preparatory stretching may include leg bends, shoulder rotations, and circular neck movements. This will help improve your functional flexibility and prevent injuries during your workout.

2. Stretching Between Exercises:

During your Pilates with Pareda practice, you can incorporate stretching between exercises. This type of stretching can help maintain your flexibility during the workout and can be particularly useful if you tend to become stiff during rest intervals. For example, after performing a set of leg exercises, you could do a light leg stretch before moving on to a core exercise.

3. Post-Workout Stretching:

After completing your Pilates with Pareda session, it's crucial to dedicate time to post-workout stretching. This type of stretching, also known as static stretching, allows you to elongate the muscles worked during the workout and gradually relax them. You can focus on specific areas of the body that may have been engaged during the workout, such as the back, legs, or shoulders. Hold each stretching position for at least 15-30 seconds to gain maximum benefits.

4. Breathing and Relaxation:

During stretching, it's essential to maintain slow and controlled breathing. Deep breathing helps relax the muscles and enhances the effectiveness of stretching. Focus on your breathing while performing stretching exercises and try to gradually relax into the movements. This mindful breathing approach will create a sense of relaxation and well-being during the process.

5. Gradual Progression:

Remember that stretching should be progressive and tailored to your individual needs. Avoid trying to force your body into extreme stretching positions, as this could lead to injuries. Instead, aim to improve your flexibility gradually over time. A qualified Pilates with Pareda instructor can provide specific guidance on which stretching exercises you should perform and how to adapt them to your fitness level.

In conclusion, effective integration of stretching into your Pilates with Pareda practice is essential for achieving optimal results and maintaining a flexible and healthy body. Make sure to include warm-up, stretching between exercises, and post-workout stretching in your routine. Mindful breathing and relaxation are key elements during the stretching process. Remember to progress gradually and listen to your body to ensure safe and effective practice.

Stretching and Relaxation

Stretching and relaxation are two closely connected elements that can greatly enrich your Pilates with Pareda practice. This chapter will explore how targeted stretching can promote muscle relaxation and mental well-being, thus contributing to a more rewarding and complete practice.

1. Muscle Relaxation:

One of the primary objectives of stretching in Pilates with Pareda is muscle relaxation. During the practice, muscles can become tense due to training and physical exertion. Targeted stretching helps release this tension, allowing muscles to gradually relax. This leads to a feeling of lightness and comfort in the body, helping to prevent the accumulation of muscle tension that can lead to stiffness and discomfort.

2. Stress and Anxiety Reduction:

Stretching provides an opportunity to reconnect with your body and carve out a moment of calm and reflection. When you focus on stretching and deep breathing, you can free yourself from stress and anxiety. The practice of Pilates with Pareda offers an ideal environment for developing mindfulness and stress reduction through stretching. This stress reduction can have a positive impact on your mental health and overall well-being.

3. Improved Body Awareness:

Stretching requires a certain level of body awareness. You need to be able to feel your muscles and tension as you perform stretching exercises. This awareness helps you identify areas of the body that may be particularly tense or stiff. Through this awareness, you can adapt your stretching exercises in a targeted manner to address your individual needs.

4. Preparation for Post-Workout Relaxation:

Post-workout stretching is a key phase for relaxing the muscles engaged during Pilates practice. This phase prepares your body for total relaxation at the end of the workout. By performing stretching and focusing on deep breathing, you can prepare your body for complete relaxation. This is especially important if you plan to dedicate time to meditation or deep relaxation after your Pilates session.

5. Overall Sense of Well-Being:

The combination of stretching and relaxation contributes to an overall sense of well-being. When your body is free from muscle tension and your spirit is relaxed, you feel lighter and more energized. This state of well-being is reflected in your posture, mindset, and disposition. It is a key aspect of Pilates with Pareda, which aims to improve your overall well-being.

In summary, stretching and relaxation are essential components of your Pilates with Pareda practice. These elements work in synergy to enhance your flexibility, reduce stress, and improve your body awareness. Through regular practice of targeted stretching and mindful relaxation, you can experience an overall sense of well-being that extends beyond your workout, enhancing the quality of your daily life.

Development of a Stretching Routine

Developing a personalized stretching routine is crucial for getting the maximum benefits from your Pilates with Pareda practice. A well-structured routine allows you to improve flexibility, prevent injuries, and increase your physical comfort. In this chapter, we will explore how you can develop a tailored stretching routine to meet your individual needs.

1. Identify Your Needs:

Before you start creating a stretching routine, it's important to identify your specific needs. Ask yourself which areas of your body might be tighter or more tense. For example, you might feel tension in your back, shoulders, or legs. By identifying these areas, you can focus your stretching routine on those parts of the body that require more attention.

2. Choose the Best Stretching Exercises:

Once you've identified the areas to address, select the most appropriate stretching exercises. In Pilates with Pareda, stretching exercises often aim to improve flexibility in the spine, shoulders, legs, and core. Some examples include the cat stretch, triceps stretch, leg stretch, and shoulder stretch. Choose exercises that best suit your needs and that you can perform safely.

3. Determine the Sequence:

The sequence in which you perform stretching exercises is important. Typically, it's advisable to start from the upper body and work your way down or vice versa. For example, you might begin with shoulder stretching exercises and then move on to leg and core stretches. This gradual flow allows your body to progressively prepare for more intense stretching.

4. Establish an Adequate Duration:

The duration of each stretching exercise should be at least 15-30 seconds to reap significant benefits. However, if you feel that you need more time to relax in a particular area or if you have chronic stiffness issues, you can extend the stretching time to 60 seconds or more. Ensure that you breathe deeply during each exercise and maintain a sense of comfort.

5. Be Consistent:

Consistency is key to achieving lasting results with your stretching routine. Try to perform your routine regularly, ideally at least three times a week. Pilates with Pareda provides an ideal opportunity to incorporate stretching into your routine, so take some time after your workout to focus on your personalized stretching.

6. Listen to Your Body:

It's crucial to listen to your body during stretching. Do not try to force your body into extreme positions or exceed your limits. Stretching should be a comfortable and relaxing experience. If you feel significant pain or discomfort, stop stretching immediately.

7. Adapt Over Time:

Over time, you may need to adapt your stretching routine based on changes in your physical needs. You may notice improvements in flexibility in some areas, while others may require more attention. Your stretching routine should be flexible and adaptable to meet these evolving needs.

In conclusion, developing a personalized stretching routine is an important step in improving flexibility, preventing injuries, and increasing your physical comfort in Pilates with

Pareda practice. Identify your needs, choose appropriate exercises, establish a suitable sequence, and be consistent in your practice. Always listen to your body and adapt your routine over time to maximize the benefits.

Chapter 8: "The Mental Side of Pilates: Balance and Mental Wellbeing"

Mindfulness and Presence

Mindfulness and presence are fundamental elements of Pilates practice with Pareda. This chapter will delve into how developing these mental skills can enhance your experience during training and your overall well-being.

Mindfulness, or awareness, is the practice of being fully present in the current moment without judgment or distraction. In the context of Pilates with Pareda, mindfulness means focusing carefully on each movement, breath, and physical sensation during training. Presence involves being fully engaged in both your body and mind while performing the exercises.

One key to developing mindfulness during Pilates is breath awareness. Breathing is the link between the mind and the body, and learning to control it is essential for improving awareness. During your practice, pay attention to the rhythm of your breath, the expansion and contraction of your chest, and the impact of breathing on each movement. Breath awareness will help you stay present and maintain control over your movements.

Mental presence during Pilates is equally important. It means concentrating on each exercise without becoming distracted or letting your thoughts wander. The practice demands constant attention to the details of movements, body positioning, and proper execution of exercises. When your mind is present, it's less likely to drift towards daily worries or stress.

Pilates with Pareda offers many opportunities to develop mindfulness and presence. Each exercise is a challenge that requires your full attention. You can start your session by focusing on your breath, establishing a slow and deep rhythm that helps you relax and enter a state of awareness. During exercises, direct your attention to how your body responds to each movement. Notice the sensation of stretching, the required strength, and core engagement.

Practising mindfulness and presence during Pilates can lead to numerous benefits. One of them is an improvement in your ability to control movements. When you are fully present, you can perform exercises with greater precision and control, which contributes to achieving better results. Furthermore, mindfulness can help reduce the risk of injuries since you are more attentive to your body's signals and less likely to force or overstrain.

Beyond physical training, mindfulness and presence can positively impact your daily life. You can apply these skills outside of the gym, enhancing your ability to manage stress, focus on work or tasks, and experience the present moment more meaningfully.

In summary, mindfulness and presence are key elements of Pilates with Pareda. Developing them requires consistent practice, but the benefits they bring to your mental and physical well-being are definitely worth it. Be present during every training session, focusing on breath and movements, and you will see how this practice positively influences your life.

Emotional Balance

Emotional balance is an essential aspect of overall well-being, and the practice of Pilates with Pareda can have a significant impact on the development of this balance. This chapter will explore how physical training, breathing, and relaxation in the context of Pilates can contribute to your emotional equilibrium.

Pilates with Pareda is much more than just a physical workout. It's an opportunity to deeply connect with your body and mind. During the training, by focusing carefully on each movement and your breath, you can create a mental space that promotes relaxation and stress management. This process can lead to greater emotional balance.

A key aspect of Pilates with Pareda is controlled breathing. Learning to breathe slowly and deeply has a calming effect on the nervous system. When you're stressed or anxious, your breathing tends to be fast and shallow. Pilates teaches you to slow down and control your breathing, which can help you relax and reduce anxiety levels. This is particularly important because breathing is one of the few bodily functions that can be consciously controlled, and you can use it to influence your emotional state.

Regular practice of Pilates with Pareda can also promote physical relaxation. Many stretching and relaxation exercises allow your muscles to gradually relax. This physical relaxation can have a direct impact on your emotional state, reducing muscle tension often associated with stress and worry.

Emotional balance is also influenced by the chemical balance in the brain. Physical exercise, including Pilates, can increase the production of neurotransmitters like endorphins and serotonin, known to improve mood and reduce the feeling of stress. Furthermore, consistent Pilates practice can lead to long-term improvements in your mental health, increasing self-esteem and self-confidence.

Pilates with Pareda can also function as a momentary escape from daily stress. During your workout session, you can temporarily step away from worries and fully focus on yourself. This can serve as a rejuvenating break for your mind, offering a sense of clarity and calm.

Finally, emotional balance is closely related to overall well-being. When you feel emotionally balanced, you are more open to new experiences, more resilient in the face of challenges, and better equipped to build meaningful relationships with others. Pilates with Pareda not only helps you achieve better emotional balance but can also positively influence other aspects of your life.

In summary, emotional balance is a valuable goal to pursue, and Pilates with Pareda provides a path to reach it. Through controlled breathing, physical relaxation, and mental focus, you can improve your emotional well-being and develop greater resilience to the stresses of daily life. Begin your Pilates practice with the goal of not only obtaining a stronger body but also a more balanced mind.

Focus and Concentration

Focus and concentration are fundamental mental skills that can be honed through the regular practice of Pilates with Pareda. This chapter will explore how to improve your focus and concentration during your workout and how these skills can positively transfer to your daily life.

Pilates with Pareda demands a high degree of concentration on every movement. Each exercise is designed to engage specific muscle groups and requires proper form and control. To perform the exercises effectively, you must be fully present, and free from distractions. This level of concentration is a hallmark of Pilates and greatly contributes to its benefits.

The practice of Pilates can be likened to a form of moving meditation. As you immerse yourself in the workout, your mind becomes free from everyday worries and focuses entirely on movements and breath. This state of "flow," or flow, is a moment of deep concentration where time seems to stand still, and all that matters is the present action. This experience can be extremely rewarding and can help you develop a greater ability to concentrate even outside of your workout.

One of the aspects that contribute to your concentration in Pilates is the coordination between the mind and the body. Exercise requires constant communication between the brain and muscles to control each movement. This improved mind-body connection can have a positive effect on your ability to concentrate on other activities, such as work or study.

The concentration developed in Pilates can also improve your short-term memory and problem-solving abilities. The mental training involved in performing exercises, following precise instructions, and adapting your body to exercise variations stimulates your mind and keeps it engaged.

Furthermore, Pilates with Pareda can teach you to approach challenges with patience and determination. Since some exercises can be demanding, they require a constant commitment to improving form and strength. This patience developed during your workout can be transferred to other life challenges, enabling you to face difficulties with greater resilience.

Finally, Pilates with Pareda provides an ideal environment to develop your concentration. Since it requires regular practice, you have the opportunity to continually work on improving your concentration skills. You can start with short sessions and gradually increase the duration and intensity of your workouts, which allows you to continuously challenge your mind and body.

In summary, focus and concentration are mental skills that can be significantly enhanced through the practice of Pilates with Pareda. The concentration required to perform exercises effectively can positively transfer to your daily life, improving your problem-solving abilities, decision-making skills, and your ability to face challenges with patience and determination. Investing time and effort in developing these skills can lead to significant improvement in your overall well-being.

Stress Management

Stress management has become a crucial component of well-being in modern society. Pilates with Pareda is a practice that can play a significant role in stress management, helping you reduce tension, regain mental calm, and improve your overall emotional state.

One of the key aspects of Pilates with Pareda is its ability to promote physical relaxation. Many of the exercises focus on stretching and relaxing muscles, helping to release accumulated bodily tension due to stress. This physical relaxation can have a direct impact on stress reduction, as tense muscles are often associated with feelings of discomfort and tension.

Controlled breathing is a fundamental element of Pilates and plays an essential role in stress management. When you're stressed, your breathing tends to be rapid and shallow. In Pilates, you learn to slow down and control your breath through specific exercises. This slowing of the breath can activate the parasympathetic nervous system, which is responsible for the body's relaxation response. By breathing deeply and in a controlled manner during your workout, you can experience an immediate reduction in stress.

Regular Pilates practice can also have a positive impact on the production of neurotransmitters in the brain. Physical exercise, including Pilates, stimulates the production of endorphins and serotonin, known to improve mood and reduce stress. These neurotransmitters act as "natural painkillers" and contribute to creating a sense of well-being and tranquillity.

Another important aspect of stress management is the ability to focus and keep the mind in the present moment. In Pilates with Pareda, each exercise requires complete concentration on movements and breathing. This concentration helps divert the mind from daily worries and keeps you focused on the present. This state of "flow" during the workout can provide you with a refreshing break from a constantly busy mind.

Physical activity in general is known for its potential to reduce stress symptoms, but Pilates has the additional advantage of being a low-impact practice. This means it is suitable for people of different ages and fitness levels, making it accessible as a stress management tool for a wide variety of individuals.

Finally, regular Pilates with Pareda practice can help you develop a sense of control in your life. When you can perform exercises with precision and control, you feel more confident in your abilities. This self-confidence can also extend to everyday life situations, helping you manage stress more effectively.

In summary, Pilates with Pareda offers a path to stress management through physical relaxation, controlled breathing, mental concentration, and the production of positive neurotransmitters. Regular training can help you develop greater emotional balance and better cope with daily challenges with calmness and determination. Investing in your Pilates practice can lead to significant improvements in your mental health and overall well-being.

Mind-Body Connection

The mind-body connection is a crucial aspect of Pilates with Pareda. This practice emphasizes the importance of uniting your mind and body during your workouts, creating a synergy that contributes to overall well-being.

In Pilates, the mind-body connection begins with awareness of movements. During each exercise, it's essential to pay attention to details, posture, and muscle control. This means you're not just performing a physical movement but also actively engaging your mind to guide and correct your body. Awareness of movements is key to achieving proper form and maximizing the benefits of your workout.

One of the unique aspects of Pilates with Pareda is the need to focus on breathing. Controlled breathing is a fundamental element of the mind-body connection. During exercises, you learn to coordinate your breath with movements, maintaining a slow and deep rhythm. This not only supplies oxygen to your muscles but also helps create a state of calm and mental focus. Breathing becomes a bridge between the body and mind, allowing for a deeper connection.

The practice of Pilates with Pareda encourages sensing and listening to your body. You learn to perceive muscle tension, strength, and comfort in various positions and movements. This physical awareness helps you identify areas that require attention and adjust your form accordingly. The mind-body connection means you're learning to listen and respond to your body's needs during your workout.

An important aspect of the mind-body connection in Pilates is the concept of "control." This means having complete control over your movements and form without overexerting yourself. The practice teaches you to perform exercises with precision, without sacrificing the quality of movement. This control helps prevent injuries and maximize the benefits of your workout.

The mind-body connection extends beyond the gym. It can positively influence other aspects of your life. For example, you become more aware of your posture and breathing in daily activities. This awareness can help reduce muscle tension and discomfort, improving your overall quality of life.

Furthermore, the mind-body connection can impact your stress management. When you're fully present during your workout, you can temporarily divert your mind from daily worries. This provides a momentary mental break and can help you relax and regain your composure.

In summary, the mind-body connection is one of the core principles of Pilates with Pareda. Through awareness of movements, controlled breathing, listening to your body, and controlling movements, you can develop a deeper connection between your mind and body. This leads to improved physical fitness, greater awareness, and enhanced overall well-being. Investing in the mind-body connection through Pilates can have a significant impact on your life, enhancing your physical and mental health.

Chapter 9: "Combating Stress and Improving Posture with Pilates"

Stress and Posture

Stress and posture are two interconnected elements that can have a significant impact on a person's overall health and well-being. In modern society, stress is a daily reality for many people and often leads to a range of physical consequences, including posture problems. In this chapter, we will explore the relationship between stress and posture and how Pilates with Pareda can play a crucial role in mitigating these negative effects.

Stress is a natural physiological response of the body to situations perceived as threatening or challenging. When you experience stress, your body releases adrenaline and other chemicals that prepare your organism to fight or flee. This reaction can cause various changes in the body, including muscle contractions.

One of the most noticeable effects of stress on posture is muscle tightening. When stressed, muscles tend to contract, especially those in the shoulder and neck area. This constant tightening can lead to chronic muscle tension and worsen posture.

People under stress often involuntarily adopt incorrect posture. They slouch their shoulders forward, round their back, and bend their neck downward. This improper posture can lead to various problems, including back pain, neck pain, and even breathing issues. Stress-influenced posture can become a perpetual cycle, as poor posture can increase discomfort, leading to more stress.

Pilates with Pareda offers an effective approach to address these issues. Pilates exercises focus on movement awareness and proper posture. During practice, you learn to relax tense muscles and correct incorrect posture. This is essential for preventing or correcting posture problems associated with stress.

Additionally, controlled breathing in Pilates plays a crucial role in stress management and posture optimization. Slowing down and controlling your breathing during exercises not only helps reduce stress but also stabilizes the spine and improves posture.

Regular Pilates practice can also strengthen core and back muscles, which are essential for maintaining an upright and correct posture. These muscles help support the spine and prevent slumping in the upper body, often associated with poor posture.

Finally, Pilates with Pareda can teach you to relax and manage stress more effectively. During practice, you learn to focus on the present, free yourself from daily worries, and connect with your body. This mental and physical awareness can help reduce tension and improve your posture in the long term.

In summary, stress and posture are linked in a vicious cycle, but Pilates with Pareda offers an effective solution to address both issues. This practice can help you relax, correct improper posture, and manage stress more effectively. Investing in your physical and mental health through Pilates can lead to better posture and an overall higher quality of life.

Exercises for Relaxation

Relaxation exercises in the context of Pilates with Pareda play a crucial role in helping you release muscle tension and improve your posture. These exercises aim to relax muscles that tend to become tense due to stress and poor postural habits. Below, we will explore some specific exercises that you can incorporate into your Pilates routine to promote body relaxation and posture improvement.

1. **Neck and Shoulder Relaxation:** This exercise is designed to relieve tension in

the neck and shoulders, which often become tense due to stress. While sitting or standing, slowly lower your chin towards your chest, then gently tilt your head to one side and then to the other. Keep the movement slow and controlled. You can also lightly rotate your head in a circle to further relax the neck. Repeat this exercise several times.

2. **Chest and Pectoral Stretch:** To relax the front of your body and improve posture, you can perform a simple chest stretch. Find a wall and stand in front of it. Place one arm on the wall at chest height and slowly rotate your body in the opposite direction. You will feel a slight stretch in the front of your chest. Hold this position for a few seconds and then switch arms.

3. **Back Relaxation:** To relax your back and improve posture, lie on your back with your knees bent and your feet flat on the floor. Extend your arms along your body with palms facing up. Take a deep breath in, and as you exhale, slowly lift your hips off the floor, pushing your feet and shoulders down. Hold this position for a few seconds, and then slowly lower your hips. Repeat the exercise several times.

4. **Leg Stretching:** To relieve tension in your legs, find an empty wall and stand about a step's distance away from it. Place your hands on the wall and extend one leg backwards while keeping the other slightly bent. You will feel a gentle stretch in the back of the extended leg. Hold the position for a few seconds and then switch legs. This exercise helps relax leg muscles and improve posture.

5. **Deep Breathing:** Controlled breathing is essential for relaxation. Sit comfortably with your back straight and your hands on your knees. Close your eyes and start to inhale slowly through your nose, counting to four. Exhale slowly through your mouth, counting to six. Focus on deep and rhythmic breathing, and try to release tension with each exhale.

These relaxation exercises can be incorporated into your Pilates with Pareda routine to help you release muscle tension and improve posture. It's important to perform them slowly and in a controlled manner, focusing on the sensation of relaxation as you do them. With regular practice, you can experience increased flexibility, reduced stress, and overall improvement in your physical and mental well-being.

Exercises for Posture

Posture exercises in the context of Pilates with Pareda are essential for improving and maintaining proper posture. Good posture not only contributes to aesthetics but also plays a key role in preventing musculoskeletal problems and reducing stress on various parts of the body. In this chapter, we will explore a series of Pilates exercises designed specifically to strengthen the muscles that support an upright and correct posture.

1. **Spinal Exercise:**

    - Sit with your legs crossed or extended in front of you.

    - Imagine elongating your spine upward, as if there's an invisible thread lifting you from the top of your head.

    - Hold this position for at least 30 seconds, focusing on the length of your spine and posture correction.

2. **Cat and Camel Exercise:**

    - Get on all fours, with hands under your shoulders and knees under your hips.

- Inhale as you slowly lift your head and tailbone upward, creating a curve in your back (Camel position).
- Exhale as you slowly roll your back upward, tucking your chin to your chest (Cat position).
- Repeat this movement smoothly for at least 1-2 minutes, focusing on spinal flexibility and posture correction.

3. **Bridge Exercise:**
   - Lie on your back with your knees bent and feet flat on the floor, hip-width apart.
   - Inhale as you slowly lift your hips upward, keeping your feet and shoulders on the ground.
   - Exhale as you slowly lower your hips.
   - Repeat this exercise at least 10-15 times to strengthen the core muscles and improve spinal stability.

4. **Chest and Deltoid Exercise:**

- Stand up and extend both arms behind you, clasping them together.
- Slowly raise your arms upward while keeping your elbows extended and palms facing each other.
- Hold this position for at least 30 seconds, feeling your chest open and the shoulder muscles engaged in posture correction.

5. **Back Straightening Exercise:**
   - Sit on a chair with your feet flat on the floor and hands placed on your hips.
   - Inhale as you lengthen your spine upward and bring your shoulders back.
   - Exhale as you gently tilt your pelvis forward, keeping your back straight.
   - Repeat this movement slowly at least 10 times to help improve sitting posture.

6. **Core Exercise:**

- Lie on your back with your knees bent and feet flat on the floor.
- Place your hands behind your head without straining your neck.
- Slowly lift your head and shoulders off the floor, contracting your abdominal muscles.
- Hold this position for a few seconds and then slowly lower your head and shoulders.
- Repeat this exercise at least 10-15 times to strengthen the core and support an upright posture.

These Pilates exercises are just a starting point for improving your posture. It's important to perform them with precision and consistency, focusing on posture correction and strengthening the key muscles that support it. Over time, proper posture will become second nature, leading to better musculoskeletal health and increased confidence in your daily posture.

Breathing and Stress

Breathing and stress are deeply interconnected. How we breathe can significantly influence our response to stress, and vice versa. In the context of Pilates with Pareda, awareness of breathing and its control is fundamental to addressing stress and improving overall well-being.

Stress is a natural body response to situations perceived as threatening or challenging. When we experience stress, the nervous system activates the "fight or flight" response, leading to an increased heart rate, blood pressure, and respiratory rate. This type of rapid and shallow breathing is effective for dealing with immediate threats but can become chronic when stress persists over time.

Pilates with Pareda offers a unique opportunity to learn to breathe more consciously and in a controlled manner. During the exercises, diaphragmatic breathing is taught, where breathing occurs through the diaphragm rather than the upper chest. This type of breathing has several key benefits:

1. **Stress Reduction:** Diaphragmatic breathing slows down the heart rate and calms the nervous system. This helps reduce physical and mental tension and stress.

2. **Increased Oxygenation:** Deep and controlled breathing allows for a greater flow of oxygen to the muscles and brain,

improving concentration and mental clarity.

3. **Core Stabilization:** Diaphragmatic breathing is crucial for core control. During Pilates exercises, you learn to coordinate breathing with movements, which helps strengthen the core muscles and improve trunk stability.

4. **Promotion of Relaxation:** Slow and deep breathing is often associated with relaxation. During Pilates, you learn to focus on your breath while performing exercises, creating a sense of calm and control.

5. **Posture Improvement:** Proper breathing supports an upright posture. This is particularly important for preventing or correcting posture problems related to stress.

Regular practice of Pilates with Pareda teaches you to integrate controlled breathing into every aspect of your daily life. You can apply this awareness of breathing not only during exercises but also when facing stressful situations outside the gym. This helps you manage stress more effectively and maintain a sense of calm and control even in intense situations.

Additionally, Pilates can help you develop greater awareness of your body and muscle tensions associated with stress. During exercises, you pay attention to the sensation of muscles contracting and relaxing. This physical awareness allows you to identify and release tension more effectively.

In summary, breathing and stress are closely connected, but Pilates with Pareda offers tools and techniques to improve breathing awareness and manage stress more effectively. Diaphragmatic breathing, body awareness, and core control become powerful tools for enhancing physical and mental well-being. Investing in your ability to breathe consciously through Pilates can lead to better stress management, improved posture, and an overall sense of balance and well-being.

Strategies for Well-being

In your journey to improve your physical and mental health through Pilates with Pareda, it's essential to implement strategies that promote long-term well-being. These strategies go beyond merely practising physical exercises and extend to your overall lifestyle. Here are some key strategies for well-being that you can integrate into your Pilates routine:

1. **Nutrient-Rich Diet:** A balanced diet is crucial to support your body in the process of strengthening and recovery after Pilates workouts. Ensure you consume a variety of nutritious foods, including fruits, vegetables, lean proteins, and whole grains. Hydration is equally important, so drink an adequate amount of water throughout the day.

2. **Adequate Rest:** Sleep is essential for your overall health and muscle recovery. Try to maintain a regular sleep routine, avoiding distractions such as electronic devices before bedtime. Adequate rest helps keep your energy levels high and reduces stress.

3. **Stress Management:** In addition to Pilates practice, consider integrating other stress management techniques into your daily life. These may include meditation, tai chi, yoga, or even simple nature walks. Find what works best for you to maintain a calm and resilient mind.

4. **Body Awareness:** Pilates is a practice that emphasizes body awareness. Bring this awareness into your daily life by paying attention to your posture, breathing, and muscle tension. This will

help you correct poor postural habits and prevent unnecessary strains.

5. **Exercise Variety:** While Pilates with Pareda is the core of your training, try to incorporate a variety of physical activities into your routine. Walk, swim, bike, or engage in other activities you enjoy. Variety helps prevent adaptation and keeps your body challenged.

6. **Social Support:** Share your Pilates experience and your goals with friends or family. Finding a support group or workout partner can be motivating and allows you to share your challenges and successes.

7. **Self-Care:** Don't forget to take care of yourself holistically. Dedicate time to activities that relax you and make you feel good, such as spending time with friends, creative hobbies, or reading a good book.

8. **Realistic Goals:** Set reasonable goals for your Pilates journey and overall well-being. Whether you're looking to improve strength, flexibility, or posture, be patient with yourself and enjoy the small progress along the way.

9. **Tracking and Assessment:** Keep a workout journal to record your progress

and goals. This allows you to track improvements over time and make any necessary adjustments to your routine.

10. **Consult a Professional:** If you have specific health concerns or pre-existing medical conditions, consult a healthcare professional, such as a physical therapist or doctor, before starting or modifying a Pilates routine.

By incorporating these strategies into your Pilates with Pareda journey, you can create a supportive environment for your physical and mental well-being. Pilates is an opportunity to develop a better awareness of your body and strengthen your physical health, but it's important to adopt a holistic approach that embraces nutrition, rest, stress management, and self-care. With a comprehensive view of well-being, you can enjoy the lasting benefits of a healthy and active life.

Chapter 10:
"Supporting an Active Lifestyle: Integrating Pilates into Your Daily Routine"

Il Pilates as a daily habit

Il Pilates as a daily habit is an effective approach to improving your physical and mental well-being in the long run. Integrating this practice into your daily routine not only helps you develop better physical fitness but also contributes to your emotional balance, body control, and proper posture. This is why Pilates should be considered not just as an occasional physical activity but as an essential habit for your well-being.

1. Body Awareness: Pilates promotes body awareness, meaning you become more attentive to the signals your body sends you. This aspect is crucial for daily well-being as it allows you to identify and address muscle tension or postural issues before they become severe. You can apply this awareness to your daily life by improving your posture while working or walking down the street.

2. Stress Management: Stress is an inevitable part of modern life, but Pilates gives you the tools to manage it more

effectively. The controlled breathing and concentration required during Pilates exercises help calm the nervous system, reduce stress, and face daily challenges with a calmer mind.

3. Posture Improvement: Many people suffer from posture problems due to long hours spent in front of the computer or sitting for extended periods. Pilates teaches you to maintain proper posture and strengthen the muscles that support it. This is crucial for preventing pain and muscle tension related to poor posture.

4. Flexibility and Mobility: Maintaining a good level of flexibility and mobility is essential for your daily health. Pilates with the Pareda helps you develop flexibility and mobility gradually and safely, which can translate into easier movement in your daily activities.

5. Core Control and Strength: Pilates is known for its focus on core control and core strength. These aspects are important not only during workouts but also in your daily activities. A strong core helps you lift objects safely, maintain stability while walking or bending, and prevent back injuries.

6. Energy and Vitality: Regular Pilates practice can increase your energy and vitality levels. This can result in higher productivity at work, better sleep quality, and an overall sense of well-being that supports you in your daily activities.

7. Long-Term Sustainability: Pilates is suitable for people of all ages and fitness levels, making it a sustainable long-term habit. You can practice it throughout your life, maintaining a good level of health and well-being even as you age.

To incorporate Pilates into your daily routine, start with small steps. You can dedicate as little as 15-20 minutes a day to Pilates exercises, perhaps in the morning or evening. Try to establish a consistent routine so that Pilates becomes a fixed appointment in your day. Over time, you'll find that this daily habit leads to significant improvements in your physical and mental health, helping you live a more active, mindful, and fulfilling life.

Moments of Awareness

Moments of awareness represent a fundamental practice for integrating Pilates into your daily routine and deriving the maximum benefit from it. These moments are based on the principle of mindfulness, which involves attention, concentration, and mindful observation of the present moment. When you apply mindfulness to Pilates and your daily life, you create a bridge between your training and your overall well-being. Here's why moments of awareness are so valuable:

1. **Breath Awareness:** One of the fundamental aspects of Pilates practice is controlled breathing. In moments of awareness, pay attention to your breath, observing how it enters and exits your body. This practice helps calm your nervous system, reduce stress, and improve your concentration.

2. **Body Awareness:** During Pilates, you develop a deep awareness of your body. In moments of awareness, extend this practice beyond the exercises. Pay attention to physical sensations, muscle tension, and daily postures. This awareness helps you identify and correct postural issues and muscle tension.

3. **Breathing Moments:** Find moments in your day for brief sessions of breathing and mindfulness. These moments can occur anywhere: while waiting in line at the grocery store, while sitting at your workplace, or before going to sleep.

Breathe deeply, focusing on the inhalation and exhalation. This helps bring your attention back to the present and reduces stress.

4. **Posture Awareness:** Moments of awareness are ideal for correcting improper posture. For example, while sitting at your desk, check the position of your back and shoulders. Correct your posture if necessary and focus your attention on the sensation of an upright posture.

5. **Active Breaks:** Transform moments of awareness into short active breaks during the day. You can perform basic Pilates exercises or simple stretching movements to relax your muscles and renew your energy. This is especially useful if you spend many hours sitting at work.

6. **Movement Awareness:** When you perform your daily activities, bring mindful attention to the quality of movement. Walk with purpose and feel the contact of your feet with the ground. Lift objects safely, engage your core muscles, and maintain proper posture. This awareness prevents sudden movements and unnecessary tensions.

7. **Experimentation:** In moments of awareness, experiment with different sensations and body movements. This is particularly helpful in understanding how Pilates principles apply to your daily life. For example, you can experiment with how core engagement supports lifting light weights or how controlled breathing influences your calmness during stressful situations.

Moments of awareness not only enhance your Pilates practice but also positively impact your daily life. They allow you to be more present in the moment, improve your posture, better manage stress, and move with increased awareness of your body. They make Pilates a comprehensive habit that goes beyond the gym and integrates into your daily life for your physical and mental well-being.

Pilates at Home

Practising Pilates at home represents an extraordinary opportunity to improve your strength, flexibility, and overall health without the need to go to a gym or fitness studio. This approach offers you the flexibility to tailor your practice to your personal needs and schedule. Here's why Pilates at home is so advantageous:

1. **Accessibility and Convenience:** Practicing Pilates at home eliminates the need for travel and fixed schedules. You can do it when and where you prefer, making your exercise routine more accessible and suitable for your lifestyle.

2. **Privacy and Comfort:** Exercising at home provides you with a private and comfortable environment. You can choose your preferred music or create a peaceful atmosphere for your practice. This allows you to feel at ease during exercises and focus on your experience without distractions.

3. **Time and Money Savings:** You don't need to pay a gym membership fee or invest in expensive equipment to practice Pilates at home. With a small initial expense for essential equipment, you'll save money in the long run and optimize your time by avoiding commuting.

4. **Customization:** Practicing at home allows you to customize your Pilates routine to your needs. You can focus on the exercises you enjoy the most or those specific to your fitness goals.

5. **Flexible Schedule:** You're not bound by gym or Pilates studio opening hours. You

can work out at dawn or midnight, depending on your schedule. This flexibility enables you to maintain a consistent practice over time.

6. **Involve Family and Friends:** Invite family members or friends to join you in practising Pilates at home. This can make your workout more fun and engaging, creating healthy competition to achieve fitness goals.

7. **Online Guidance and Resources:** With internet access, you have a wide range of online resources to guide you in practising Pilates at home. You can find video tutorials, step-by-step guides, and specific training programs. These resources help you perform exercises correctly and safely.

8. **Personal Progress:** Keeping a workout journal allows you to track your progress over time. You can record details of your sessions, including exercises performed and repetitions, to assess improvements in your fitness level.

9. **Increased Body Awareness:** Practicing at home gives you the opportunity to develop a greater awareness of your body. You can focus on listening to muscle

sensations and strengthening the mind-body connection during exercises.

10. **Routine Maintenance:** When you have Pilates equipment at home, you are more likely to maintain a consistent routine. This is essential for achieving lasting results over time.

To get started with Pilates at home, you'll need some basic equipment like a mat, a Pareda (The Wall), or a stable chair. You can find online video tutorials or invest in virtual lessons with certified Pilates instructors to guide you in your practice. With commitment and consistency, Pilates at home can become a valuable component of your wellness routine, delivering both physical and mental benefits.

Involving Family and Friends

Involving family and friends in your Pilates practice is a great strategy to make your workouts more enjoyable, motivating, and socially engaging. This approach not only allows you to share the benefits of Pilates with your loved ones but also creates a supportive environment that enhances your commitment and consistency in your practice. Here's why involving family and friends is so important:

1. **Sharing Experiences:** By involving your loved ones in Pilates practice, you have the opportunity to share meaningful experiences together. This creates stronger bonds and enables you to support each other in your wellness journeys.

2. **Motivation:** Exercising with friends or family can significantly boost motivation. Knowing that there are others expecting you to participate in the workout can give you the push you need to maintain consistency in your practice.

3. **Fun:** Pilates can be a fun activity to share with others. You can do exercises together, joke around, and laugh during the workout. This makes the experience more enjoyable and less monotonous.

4. **Mutual Support:** When facing similar fitness challenges or goals, you can offer each other valuable mutual support. Discuss your progress, achievements, and challenges, creating an environment of understanding and encouragement.

5. **Personal Growth:** By involving others in your Pilates practice, you can contribute to their personal growth and well-being. You can share your knowledge,

experiences, and techniques for improving posture, strength, and flexibility.

6. **Strengthening Family Bonds:** Pilates practice can become a special time to spend with your family. It's an opportunity to create positive memories and strengthen family bonds through a shared activity.

7. **Variation in Workouts:** Involving family and friends can lead to variations in the types of exercises and routines. Everyone can bring in new ideas and perspectives, creating a richer and more interesting practice.

8. **Developing Healthy Habits:** Involving your loved ones in Pilates practice helps develop healthy habits within your social circle. This can positively influence their overall approach to fitness and well-being.

9. **Shared Accountability:** When you have a workout partner, you share a sense of accountability. This motivates you to keep commitments and maintain a more consistent Pilates routine.

10. **Personal Satisfaction:** Seeing your loved ones benefit from Pilates practice can give

you a deep sense of personal satisfaction. You know that you've positively contributed to their health and well-being.

To involve family and friends in Pilates, you can organize home workout sessions, participate in group classes together, or commit to following online fitness programs as a group. It's important to tailor the practice to the needs and fitness levels of each participant and ensure that it's a positive and enjoyable experience for everyone. Ultimately, involving others in your Pilates journey creates a supportive and sharing environment that enriches your practice and strengthens social bonds.

Maintain Variety

Maintaining variety in your Pilates practice is a fundamental strategy for achieving lasting results and keeping it interesting over time. Changing exercises, modes, and approaches challenges your body in different ways, prevents boredom and avoids hitting a plateau where your body gets accustomed to a routine and stops progressing. Here's why variety is so crucial in your Pilates practice:

1. **Constant Stimulation:** Changing Pilates exercises and routines constantly

stimulates your body. This prevents your muscular and nervous systems from adapting too quickly, allowing for continuous improvements in strength, flexibility, and control.

2. **Target Different Body Parts:** Variety allows you to target different parts of your body specifically. You can focus on different muscle groups or specific goals, such as core strengthening, spinal flexibility, or posture improvement.

3. **Injury Prevention:** Repeating the same movements continuously can increase the risk of overuse injuries. Variety reduces this risk by distributing muscle and joint usage more evenly.

4. **Sustain Interest:** Variety keeps your interest alive in your Pilates practice. When sessions become boring, you are less likely to engage enthusiastically. Trying out new exercises and approaches can renew your interest and motivation.

5. **Fitness Level Adaptation:** Variety lets you adapt your practice to your fitness level. You can start with basic exercises and gradually progress to more advanced ones as you become stronger and more flexible.

6. **Greater Mental Benefits:** Varying your Pilates practice can also lead to mental benefits. You can develop greater concentration and awareness when performing new movements and challenges.

7. **Deepen Understanding:** Experimenting with different Pilates exercises helps you better understand how your body works. You learn how various muscles and joints interact and how you can use them more efficiently.

8. **Creativity and Fun:** Trying out new exercises gives you the opportunity to explore your creativity and make your Pilates practice fun. You can customize your routine based on your preferences and specific needs.

9. **Continuous Progress:** By maintaining variety, you can continuously progress toward your fitness goals. You can set short-term and long-term goals and work toward them through new challenges and exercises.

10. **Adaptability:** Variety makes you more adaptable to different situations. You can easily incorporate Pilates into other aspects of your life, such as sports or

work because you've developed a wide range of physical and mental abilities.

To maintain variety in your Pilates practice, you can explore new exercises, participate in group classes with experienced instructors, use different equipment like the Pareda or Pilates ball, and incorporate other forms of fitness into your routine. The key is to be open to exploration and experimentation so that you can reap the maximum benefits from your Pilates practice in the long run.

Conclusion

As we come to the end of this journey through the world of "Wall Pilates," it's important to reflect on what we've learned and how we can apply this knowledge to our daily lives. "Wall Pilates" is much more than a simple exercise system; it's a path to strengthening the body and mental well-being, leading us to a state of extraordinary and lasting health. In this conclusion, we will examine the key teachings we have acquired and how we can continue to thrive through this innovative approach to Pilates.

Synthesis of the Fundamental Principles of Pilates

First and foremost, it is crucial to remember the fundamental principles of Pilates that have accompanied us throughout the book. Concentration, control, precision, breath, and fluidity of movement are the building blocks of Pilates practice. These principles not only shape our bodies but also help us develop a deeper connection between mind and body. By continuing to honour these principles, we can ensure that every wall Pilates session is an opportunity to enhance our awareness, strength, and inner balance.

The Central Role of the Wall

The wall has been our most precious ally on this journey. It provided support, stability, and limitless movement possibilities. "Wall Pilates" has demonstrated that an apparently static element can become a dynamic tool for muscle strengthening and flexibility improvement. The wall is a symbol of unconditional support, just as our bodies must become for ourselves. By continuing to harness the potential of the wall, we can reach new heights of strength and well-being.

Continuous Progress

One of the most important teachings of this book is that progress in "Wall Pilates" is an ongoing process. No matter where you start from, with consistency and dedication, you can improve your strength, flexibility, and overall health. Each Pilates session represents an opportunity to grow and progress. We should never stop challenging ourselves and seeking to surpass our limits because that's where real transformation begins.

Balancing Body and Mind

Pilates is much more than a simple physical exercise. It's a complete experience that teaches us to balance body and mind. During each session, we've learned to focus on our breath, develop awareness of our body, and control our movements precisely. These teachings can be applied not only to Pilates practice but also to our daily lives. When we can achieve a balance between body and mind, we can face challenges with greater calmness and determination.

Consistent Practice as the Key to Success

Finally, it's essential to remember that success in "Wall Pilates" requires consistent practice. To reap the maximum benefits from this form of training, we must commit to maintaining a regular routine. It doesn't matter how short or challenging the session is; what matters is consistency. Over time, the results will become evident, and we'll realize that our investment in our health was worth it.

In conclusion, "Wall Pilates" represents an extraordinary gateway to strengthening the body and lasting well-being. It's a path that can transform our lives in ways that go far beyond physical benefits. It teaches us to connect with ourselves, cultivate mental strength, and create a solid foundation upon which to build a healthy and fulfilling life. By continuing to honour the principles of Pilates, harnessing the potential of the wall, and committing to consistent practice, we can achieve extraordinary levels of strength and lasting well-being that will accompany us for the rest of our lives. The key lies in taking action, starting the journey, and persevering with determination. "Wall Pilates" is the gateway that opens to a future of extraordinary strength and lasting well-being. Now is the time to begin your journey.

Printed in the USA
CPSIA information can be obtained
at www.ICGtesting.com
LVHW010649020124
767898LV00009B/488